Bearing the Weight of the World

Exploring Maternal Embodiment

EDITED BY
ALYS EINION
AND JEN RINALDI

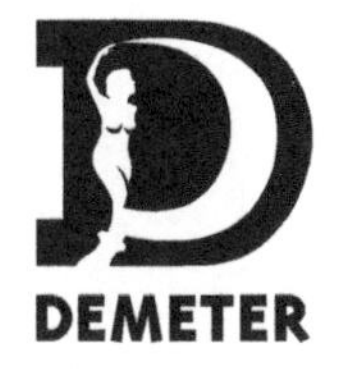

Bearing the Weight of the World
Exploring Maternal Embodiment

Edited by Alys Einion and Jen Rinaldi

Demeter Press
140 Holland Street West
P. O. Box 13022
Bradford, ON L3Z 2Y5
Tel: (905) 775-9089
Email: info@demeterpress.org
Website: www.demeterpress.org

Demeter Press logo based on the sculpture "Demeter" by Maria-Luise Bodirsky
www.keramik-atelier.bodirsky.de

Printed and Bound in Canada

Front cover image "Morgan's Birth" 40"X 30 " Oil on Canvas self-portrait
© 2001 Karen Walasek, MFA
Cover design and typesetting Michelle Pirovich

Library and Archives Canada Cataloguing in Publication
Bearing the weight of the world : exploring maternal embodiment / edited by Alys Einion and Jen Rinaldi.
Includes bibliographical references.
ISBN 978-1-77258-171-3 (softcover)
1. Motherhood--Social aspects. 2. Human body--Social aspects.
I. Einion, Alys, 1970-, editor II. Rinaldi, Jen, 1983-, editor

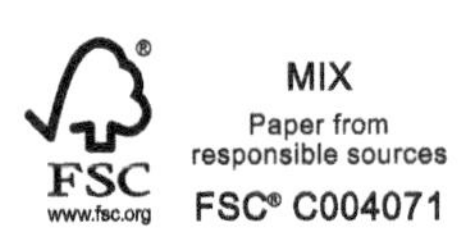

Alys:
To my sons, Gwythyr Arawn Einion, without whom I would never have become a midwife, and Aran Mortimer Henley-Einion, my pride and my joy, who showed me how to be a mother.

Jen:
To my mother, who supports me; and my father, who was proud of me

Contents

Foreword

Alys Einion

This book has been a long time in coming to life. It grew from the smallest seed of an idea that women remain caught up in a constant battle to occupy their own space in the world and in the wondrous and powerful bodies that house us. There have been many books and articles written about the power dynamics of pregnancy, birth, and childbearing, the unrealistic expectations on women's bodily shape, size, and behaviour, and the inequalities of medical hegemonic power within the domain of childbearing. Women, professionals, and practitioners have become increasingly aware of the multiple ways in which bodily autonomy is eroded and respect for women is erased. This volume was meant to show that women are powerfully present in current debates around childbearing and embodied experience and that our voices should be the first to be heard.

There is much to be learned from hearing and sharing mothers' knowledge. There are different perspectives and experiences to enlighten us and stimulate reflection and conversation. But most of all, there is a continuing need for a corpus of critical-creative work that not only adds to the childbearing canon but actively encourages women to own their stories, intuitive knowledge, and strength, which all come from simply living, surviving, and thriving in this world. I hope this volume gives voice to some of the multi-tonal maternal harmonies continuing to resonate around the globe. We are all unique, but in the experience of mothering we are united. It is in our commonality as much as in our individuality that we will locate the seeds for a future world of greater reproductive and personal freedom.

Swansea, United Kingdom, 2018.

Introduction

Bearing the Weight of the World: Exploring Maternal Embodiment

Alys Einion and Jen Rinaldi

A mother's body is a site of contested dynamics of power, identity, experience, autonomy, and control. Representations of the maternal body can often mis/represent the childbearing and mothering form as monstrous, idealized, limited, scrutinized, or occupied. The maternal body has long been a hypervisible artifact: at once absent from historical characterizations of pregnancy emphasizing the contributions of sperm carriers or fetal status, and a target of political, social, and medical hostility and suspicion. Readings of the maternal body as out of control justify surveillance mechanisms, medical scrutiny, expert advice, commodification, censure, and expectation of self-discipline. Thus, mothering bodies are subject to significant oversight, judgment, criticism, political- and health-oriented control systems, and culturally constructed expectations. In and through these discursive frames and practices, corporeal boundaries are produced, contained, and displaced.

Alternative accountings of embodiment and embodied resistance, however, remain underresearched and underrepresented (Parry 786; Thurer). The materiality of maternal experience, and its centrality to family and social life, remains too often viewed as a fringe subject—the province of feminists and activists, so-called hysterical women. This is despite the centuries of social and political activism that has sought to enshrine women's rights, reproductive rights, and bodily freedoms in law and in reality. The advice and scientific opinion shaping understandings of women's bodies over time is not without bias (Ehrenreich and English xiv).

In *Bearing the Weight of the World: Exploring Maternal Embodiment,* contributors explore and expose key debates around maternal embodiment from a range of disciplines—including health, art, science, law, and sociocultural studies—as well as from personal experience. This critical-creative work encompasses new insights and research that combine the personal and the pervasive, and it points to new meaning-making in critical motherhood studies via the medium of the maternal body. The academic and creative contributions enclosed countenance the maternal body and the bodily experience of pregnancy, birth, and motherhood in an analysis foregrounding embodiment as an affective medium and a site of value.

What counts as maternal is myriad. In this collection, chapters showcase a range of experiences and processes related to pregnancy. Contributors explore the ways pregnant bodies are regarded and treated, and the ways pregnant bodies develop, operate, and resist. They also consider the choreography of birthing: its moments of pain, beauty, transformation, and loss. Yet bodies are not maternal only through pregnancy, and, therefore, this collection also considers breastfeeding and beyond. Thus, contributors tend to position the maternal body in relation to reproductive function. They also tend to frame their analysis in gendered terms, referencing and prioritizing women and female experience. Although these parameters speak to our scope, we recognize that motherhood, and thus the mother's body, extends beyond pregnancy, childbirth, and breastfeeding and that the experiences of pregnancy, childbirth, and breastfeeding are not unique to women but are accessible to and experienced by trans men and genderqueer and gender-nonconforming folk.

What does it mean to be embodied? Alexandra Howson describes it as follows: "the physical characteristics of our own bodies, our mannerisms, shape, size, habits and movements, contribute to and shape our perceptions and interactions with others in everyday life" (2). We are embodied selves. Therefore, embodiment means seeing "the world and operate within it from the particular vantage-point of our own body" (Howson 2). The legacy of the Cartesian distinction between mind and body suggests a fracturing of self: the mind is self, and the body is the tool of self. Embodiment focuses more on the lived experience of the self, which includes the relationship with the body and the body's relationship with the wider world (Howson 214). The embodied self, and in particular the female self, could be argued to enact its reproductive, so-called natural functions within the private sphere of the home, the locus of motherhood (Martin 16). However, increasingly, the representation of embodied motherhood found in the public sphere suggests that these functions and activities are no longer private.

Background

Women powerfully embody the negotiation between the two theoretical standpoints—the body as "biological phenomenon" and "the social constructionist view of the body as infinitely malleable" (Shilling 17). Patriarchal social relations subordinate women by distorting the female body (Shilling 63) and by conceptualizing women in relation to their bodies, and then subjecting those bodies to violation and abuse. As Margrit Shildrick argues, "women are supposedly rooted in base corporeality.... And it is this supposed immanence that provides the justification ... for the exclusion of women from the attribute of full rationality, which is one of the essential parameters of moral agency" (81). If women are only bodies, so the logic goes, then they lack the moral agency necessary for full personhood, for equal status, and, thus, for their own decision making. In a similar vein, Elizabeth Grosz describes how women's corporeal grounding has served to justify their subordination: "patriarchal oppression ... justifies itself ... by connecting women much more closely than men to the body and, through this identification, restricting women's social and economic roles to (pseudo) biological terms" (14).

Nowhere is this more evident than in the maternal body, which is subdued, monitored, controlled and subjected to the control and interference of so-called experts (Ehrenreich and English xii). The maternal body disrupts the notion of a unified, ideal body, as the bleeding, bloating, and lactating maternal body is unruly, unstable, and messy. Rebecca Kukla describes the implications: "mothers [have historically been] implored to develop self-control and self-discipline in order to compensate for their vulnerable and poorly bounded bodies" (85). At the same time, as Barbara Katz Rothman shows, the holistic maternal experience has been subverted, supplanted, and interrupted via technological means (23). Thus, breastfeeding has become unnecessary (and taboo), birth can be accomplished surgically, and even carrying the child to full term is no longer required (Katz Rothman 23). Susan Bordo describes women's bodies as "the locus of practical cultural control" (183), which derives from the perception of the "female subject as dominated by the demands of her body" (Lupton and Schmied 829). Women are discounted as experts on their own bodies.

Women, and especially mothers, then, are known as and through limited understandings of their bodily reality. Patriarchal forces interpret maternal identity formation in relation to pervasive narratives of self-denial, control, and unrealistic expectation of body size and presentation (Roth et al. 128). Social valuing has poorly articulated the joy, wonder, and pleasure of childbearing and parenthood, as well as the work needed to adapt to the changes and identity transitions (Redshaw and Martin 305). The postnatal period—far from being a time of bonding and connection with the infant (Orbach and Rubin)—is in fact a time that establishes "mothering, beauty and body work as the most important components of maternal femininity" (Hallstein 116). The turbulent waters of transitional identity are negotiated through the lens of social scrutiny and, thus, miss the emergent relationship between mother and infant. Little recognition is given to the immense physical and emotional drain that mothers experience, or to their constant anxiety caused by the societal parameters of good mothering.

We do not counter these narrow readings of the body by separating persons from their bodies or by reconceptualizing identity and personhood as abstracted from bodies. What is needed instead is more encompassing and compassionate theorizing around embodiment. Such theorizing may frame embodiment as awareness of the privileging of mind over body in the modern period, as described by David Nikkel, and the limitations of such a philosophical standpoint for understanding women's experience of motherhood. This awareness may reckon with how "a person always stands embodied, enmeshed, enculturated in meaning and value" (Nikkel 6). Thus, the perspectives on embodiment explored in this collection advocate for a greater understanding of the subjective experience of the physical and social dimensions of pregnancy, birth, and parenting, while accepting that even the ways that we discuss this issue remain culturally conditioned (Nikkel 6). This book considers multiple voices but does not claim any as *the* voice, or as an absolute truth. Hence, we combine the critical with the personal, the creative with the academic, to better celebrate diversity of experience and offer the reader greater scope for finding some reflection of their own experience within these pages.

Chapter Outline

In "Maternal Surveillance, Maternal Control: The Paradox of the Childbearing Body," Alys Einion uses her perspective as a midwife and a mother to explore the way surveillance and medicalization of childbearing affects women's experience of pregnancy, birth, and motherhood. Referencing the concepts of bodily control and regulation, and exploring the relationship between medicine, power, and disempowerment, she discusses the assumption of Western society that medicine knows best. She argues against the separation of self from pregnancy, and suggests that the typical birth script characterizes doctors and midwives as powerful saviours and women as weaker victims in need of saving. She mounts a feminist critique of women's disempowerment through their bodily realities and the institutional control of specialist knowledge surrounding pregnancy and birth. Drawing on her own lived experience as a mother and her professional experience and research, she argues that the fundamental social construction of gender requires women to perform motherhood in limited ways. She exhorts women, midwives, and doctors to resist essentializing pregnancy and childbearing, to challenge the institutionalized control of women's bodies, and to return the power and control to those who experience pregnancy and parenting.

In their chapter "Dangerous Bodies: Imagining, Monitoring, and Managing Fatness during Pregnancy," Megan Davidson and Sarah Lewin challenge the dominant discourses of health and criticize the hidden agenda and the value base of health-oriented approaches to obesity. Highlighting how fatness has been demonized in both media and health debates, as well as the coding of fatness as risky, selfish, and irresponsible, they wish to reclaim pregnancy and childbearing, and strive for the freedom to be pregnant without body size judgment. They highlight the limitations of the evidence base relating to larger body size and pregnancy risks, and argue for resistance and a reconceptualization of the moral value of female body size. They suggest that fatphobia increases the risks and rates of medical intervention in pregnancies when the woman does not adhere to the socially accepted body shape.

In "'Consideration of the Unborn Child': Advance Directives and Pregnancy Exclusion Laws," Claire Marguerite Leonard Horn analyzes American statutory and case law, with a focus on *Munoz v. John Peter Smith Hospital*, to defend pregnant women's right to die when declared braindead. Horn invokes examples of women subjected to life-sustaining measures despite advanced directives, loved ones' demands, and fetal development falling short of viability. Her Foucauldian analysis demonstrates that pregnancy exclusions in right-to-die law reflect state control over maternal bodies.

In "Manufacturing the Mother: Technical Appropriations of Birth in Ancient Greek Thought," Jessica Elbert Decker examines the power of myths that exert male power over the female body and its natural processes of reproduction. She links Western patriarchal tropes of control to current paradigms and philosophies undermining women's bodily autonomy. Her analysis of three familiar myths illustrates the denigration of the female body common in these stories and the female body's alignment with uncontrolled nature. She argues for work that challenges the legacy of such narratives, which are still found in discourses of objectivity and reproductive control.

In "Seeding the Future: Maternal Microbiome as Maternal Embodiment," Rebecca Howes-Mischel considers how maternal embodiment comes to matter and materialize in studies of vaginal microbiomes as reported in peer-reviewed and popular scientific sources. She argues that current scientific studies clustered around microbiological risk to fetal post-genomic outcome at once elide and implicate the maternal body. Specifically, the vaginal environment is rendered ecosystemic, a conduit of intergenerational microbial relation. In a telling example, the documentary *Microbirth* portrays maternal responsibility as bodily mediated, at the microbiological level.

Ruchika Wason Singh produces artistic works while reflecting on her artistic practice in "The Temporality of Maternal Embodiment and the Creative Process: Project *Transit Spaces*." In red and pink hues, spongy objects hover within their frames, spotted with what appear to be light in one depiction, seeds in another. Plantlike branches sprout and stretch across the canvasses. Not overtly anything, these amorphous objects represent something like interior growth. Singh considers how these works were produced during her pregnancy, designed to convey vegetative force and transitory movement. The work is fleshy through and through—the colour of tissue and sinew, and of coursing, pulsing blood. The growth of pregnancy, here, is inextricable from mother flesh.

Erynne M. Gilpin and Sarah Marie Wiebe craft a decolonial analysis connecting environmental and reproductive justice in "Embodied Governance: Community Health, Indigenous Self-Determination, and Birth Practices." They propose a governance model drawing on Indigenous principles—women leadership as well as kinship relationality regarding Land as body and Water as blood—to counter colonial uses of Land and Water, which they hold stand in integral relation to the maternal body. Their proposal seeks to resituate pregnancy and labour in community and on homeland.

In "Indeterminate Life: Dealing with Radioactive Contamination as a Voluntary Evacuee Mother," Maxime Polleri discusses the aftermath of the 2011 earthquake and tsunami that resulted in catastrophic damage to the Fukishima Daiichi Nuclear Power Plant in Japan and the subsequent radioactive contamination. Presenting the stories and voices of the mothers whose lives and children have been affected by this disaster, Polleri explores the embodiment of contamination and uses agential realism to examine the symbolic relationship of contamination between self and environment. By focusing on self-evacuee mothers, the gendered nature of risk, and the wider and long-term impact of contamination, Polleri argues that mothers' concerns for their children can be viewed as oppositional to state-sanctioned information, and can reveal maternal inequality and structural injustice.

In "The Limitations and Possibilities of Genetic Imagery," Jen Rinaldi challenges the geneticized logics influencing interpretations of the chromosomal imagery yielded from disability de-selective prenatal screening procedures, specifically amniocentesis and chorionic villus sampling. She works to turn genetic deterministic interpretations of this imagery on their head through use of materialist feminist analysis, which posits that matter carries agential capacity. This chapter's feminist fashioning of epigenetics recentres the maternal body as a site of creative force.

Carla Ionescu contemplates the power of monstrous and divine depictions of breastfeeding in "Feeding the World: Reconsidering the

Multibreasted Body of Artemis Ephesia." Mother goddess figure Artemis Ephesia was frequently depicted in Ancient Greek sculpture with emphasized reproductive features, especially with many breasts. These imposing, often largescale works of a goddess carrying many variations and titles, according to Ionescu, demonstrated in material and imagery strong ties to the earth and fertility. Although this imagery scandalized Christians (despite some thematic through lines being passed onto iconography of the Virgin Mary), Ionescu suggests it is possible to find political and spiritual force in these representations of maternal embodiment.

In "'I'm MY Breastfeeding Expert': How First-Time Mothers Reclaimed their Power through Breastfeeding," Catherine Ma explores the impact of the biomedical model on the experiences of first-time mothers learning to breastfeed. She argues against the dominant practices of the biomedical model of maternity care, which negatively affect the physiological responses promoting breastfeeding. Her findings illuminate mothers' understanding of their infants' active involvement in breastfeeding and their growing confidence in their intuitive self-knowledge of feeding over time. The reclamation of being an expert on her breastfeeding shows the mother as engaging in empowering maternal transformations.

Laura Major's chapter, "Muriel Rukeyser: 'In the Body's Ghetto,'" highlights the work of a poet, Rukeyser, who has presented a reimagining of self, embodiment, pregnancy, and birth that is both critically real and linguistically and artistically distinctive. Rukeyser's groundbreaking, often invisible body of work explores the experiences of pregnancy by engaging with self and fetus, pregnant self and material child. Major explores the relationship of her work to mythological re-envisioning located within the symbolism of the female embodied self.

"Freedom to Labour—A Case Study on Childbirth Education and the Creation of Medical Choreographies" by Katie Nicole Stahl-Kovell, is a treatise on the physicality of labour. Stahl-Kovell argues against the use of linear logic and for an understanding of birth knowledge enactment in her exploration of the ethnically constituted inequalities of childbirth experience in California. She uses the term "choreo-policing" to describe how women's compliance is managed by healthcare providers during labour and birth and how the use of birth preparation classes reinforces the birthing woman's dependence on (and resistance to) medical authority. Critical dance studies, though, places the woman as a creative choreographer, often through improvisation, of her own birth experience in response to embodied knowledge.

This volume adds to the knowledge and insights about embodied experiences of maternity and the forms of identity construction that occur during this transition period mediated by specific social forces. The voices contained herein represent diverse and unique perspectives, while echoing common concerns and understandings. As Elena Neiterman shows, women are "doing" pregnancy (and motherhood) in ways that are powerfully affected by social acceptance, trends, and validation (372). We can only grow in power through understanding these varied experiences and by valuing the specialist knowledge that comes from the lived experience of mothering.

As mothers, we step into each day of our lives as explorers of new territory. We wear the familiar masks of womanhood, femininity, motherhood, and self, and we negotiate new paths through distressingly familiar territory. This territory is a landscape of peaks and troughs, beauty and pitfalls. We are furnished with imperfect maps of knowing, dim lights of understanding, and broken compasses—all ineffective tools for working our way through this perilous, wondrous land of motherhood. *Bearing the Weight of the World,* we hope, will shine a path through this motherland, signposting the way for others. We hope it will provide greater knowledge and trust in self—in the integrated self, both embodied and empowered.

Works Cited

Bordo, Susan. *Unbearable Weight: Feminism, Western Culture and the Body.* University of California Press, 2003.

Ehrenreich, Barbara, and Deirdre English. *For Her Own Good.* Anchor Books, 1978.

Grosz, Elizabeth. Volatile Bodies: Toward a Corporeal Feminism. Indiana University Press, 1994.

Hallstein, Lynn O'Brien. "She Gives Birth, She's Wearing a Bikini: Mobilizing the Postpregnant Celebrity Mom Body to Manage the Post-Second Wave Crisis in Femininity."

Women's Studies in Communication, vol. 34, no. 2, 2011, pp. 172-75.

Howson, Alexandra. *The Body in Society*. Polity Press, 2004.

Katz Rothman. *Recreating Motherhood.* Rutgers University Press, 2000.

Kukla, Rebecca. *Mass Hysteria: Medicine, Culture, and Mothers' Bodies.* Rowman and Littlefield Publishers, Inc., 2005.

Lupton, Deborah, and Virginia Schmied. "Splitting Bodies/Selves: Women's Concepts of Embodiment at the Moment of Birth." *Sociology of Health and Illness*, vol. 25, no. 6, 2012, pp. 828-41.

Martin, Emily. *The Woman in the Body*. Open University Press, 1989.

Neiterman, Elena. "Doing Pregnancy: Pregnant Embodiment as Performance." *Women's Studies International Forum*, vol. 35, 2012, pp. 372-83.

Nikkel, David H. *Radical Embodiment*. James Clark and Co., 2011.

Orbach, Susie, and Holli Rubin. "Two for the Price of One: The Impact of Body Image during Pregnancy and after Birth." *Maternal Mental Health Alliance*, 2012, maternalmentalhealthalliance.org/wp-content/uploads/Susie-Orbach-and-Holli-Rubin-Two-for-the-Price-of-One.pdf. Accessed 17 July 2018.

Parry, Diana C. "'We Wanted a Birth Experience, Not a Medical Experience': Exploring Canadian Women's Use of Midwifery." *Health Care for Women International*, vol. 29, no. 8-9, 2008, pp. 785-806.

Redshaw, Maggie, and Colin Martin. "Motherhood: A Natural Progression and a Major Transition." *Journal of Reproductive and Infant Psychology*, vol. 29, no. 4, 2011, pp. 305-7.

Roth, Heike, et al. "'Bouncing Back.' How Australia's Leading Women's Magazines Portray the Postpartum 'Body.'" *Women and Birth*, vol. 25, no. 3, 2012, pp. 128-34.

Shildrick, Margrit. *Embodying the Monster: Encounters with the Vulnerable Self.* Sage Publications, 2001.

Shilling, Chris. *The Body and Social Theory*. Sage Publications, 1993.

Thurer, Shari L. *The Myths of Motherhood: How Culture Reinvents the Good Mother.* Houghton Mifflin Company, 1994.

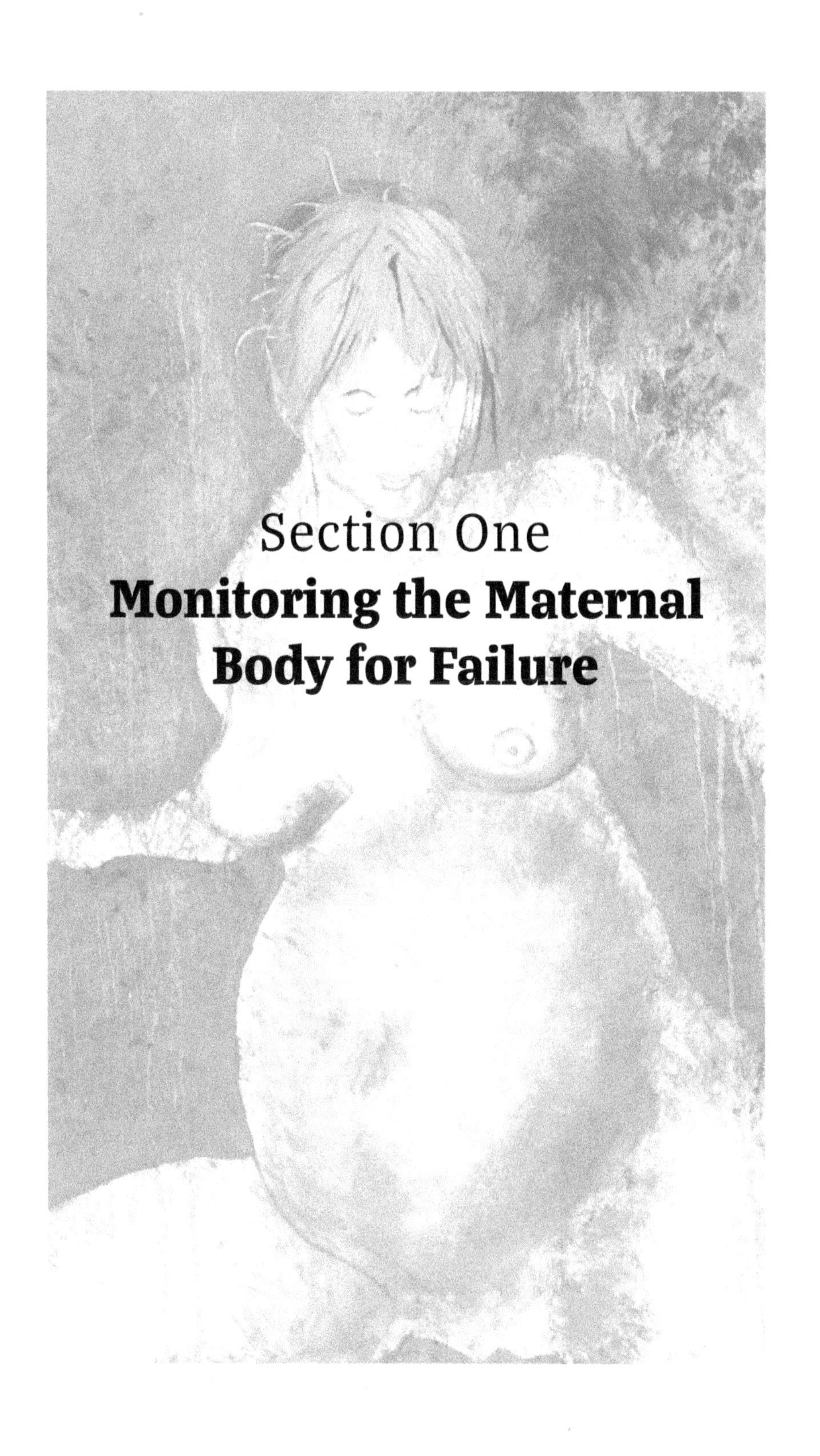

Section One
Monitoring the Maternal Body for Failure

Chapter One

Maternal Surveillance, Maternal Control: The Paradox of the Childbearing Body

Alys Einion

Ringing bells, running feet, the swish and clunk of doors opening and closing, the hiss of the Entonox, the moan and sigh of the birthing woman. The smells of chemicals and sweat and body fluids, the intense frown on the mother's face, the sudden first cry of a newborn. The smiles, the joy, the relief, breathing out, crying, the rattle of the computer keyboard, the triumphant tick on the communications board, mother and baby safe and well.

Working as a midwife for twenty years certainly sharpens one's awareness of the context in which birthing takes place—one characterized by the dichotomy between the power of innate nature and the assertions of science, an uneasy marriage of opposites. Drawing on my experience, service evaluations, and research, this chapter focuses on medical surveillance of maternal bodies within Westernized medical spaces, particularly the UK and North America, before, during, and after reproduction.

Childbearing represents a force for radical change across the life course—not just in relation to the physical experience of pregnancy, birth, and breastfeeding, but in relation to the adaptation of the woman's identity to socially constructed and embodied dimensions of motherhood. Women who choose to bear children, however, are subject to an ideology, represented in popular media, health discourse, and research, that conceptualizes childbearing as a period when women do not have control over their bodies (Carter).

The great irony of this dominant discourse is that it is during this time that "women are also subject to a cultural mandate to assume control over bodily functions through the notion of individual responsibility for fetal outcomes" (Carter 993). This sense of responsibility permeates parents' awareness of their childbearing journey, and precipitates the fear of something going wrong. This fear enables technocratic medicine to exert its control over women's bodies. This concept of bodily control and self-regulation, perpetuated by the discourses of childbearing within maternity services and healthcare, promotes the Cartesian dualism of seeing the body as separate from the self and as something to be regulated and managed according to culturally determined expectations of pregnancy, birth, and motherhood.

The body has been constructed throughout history as separate from the self. The nonphysical self is seen as something spiritual or holy, whereas the body is seen as something base and, by implication, unholy (Bordo 5). Women's bodies are subject to more overt connections with primordial physical changes—including menstruation, childbearing, and breastfeeding—and, thus, are associated with some kind of lesser state than the male body, which is seen as less wild and changeable. As Susan Bordo states, "if, whatever the specific historical content of the duality, *the body* is the negative term, and if the woman *is* the body, then women *are* that negativity, whatever it may be: distraction from knowledge, seduction away from God, capitulation to sexual desire, violence or aggression, failure of will, even death" (emphasis in original, 5).

This discourse is founded in a Westernized medical and scientific paradigm in which women's bodies are still viewed as inferior, base, natural, and out of control, and within which the dominance of fashion-driven views of body shape and size continues to underpin the limited science and research into women's health. Despite the work carried out in Western feminism to challenge the ways our culture perpetuates unrealistic ideals of women's bodies and to understand the nature of female embodiment, viewing the female body as both requiring and eminently subject to control continues to be perpetuated through one of society's most powerful institutions: medicine.

I have witnessed this discourse in my experience of working with childbearing women and families, and in particular, in my recent experience providing antenatal classes in hypnotic relaxation and birth preparation. I have experienced women entering my classes visibly terrified and unbearably tense in anticipation of their approaching birth. One source of this tension is the local midwife-run antenatal preparation classes, funded by the National Health Services (NHS). The disassociation between self and body and the impending loss of control and the promise of suffering are apparent. One client described a midwife in an NHS class who passed a pair of obstetric forceps around the room, and apparently said "one in four of you will need these." No explanation of this supposed chance was given, and no discussion of ways to enhance the physiology of birth and reduce the need for medical assistance was offered. This example, which was confirmed independently and spontaneously by other colleagues, runs in direct opposition to the discourse of control, choice, and empowerment underpinning the philosophy of midwifery and enshrining women's fundamental rights in childbearing, rights that far too few women are aware of. In my private hypnobirthing classes, I have moved from my initial ideal of helping women cope with the physical realities of childbirth through deep relaxation techniques to focusing on informed choice, autonomy, and childbearing rights to enable women and partners to challenge the dominant ideology of the birthing room.

It is impossible to consider maternal embodiment and surveillance of the childbearing body without deconstructing the dimensions of the debates around choice, control, and the ideologies of birthing. At the very basic level, this relates to the nature of gender within Western society and the fact that bodies are gendered. Considering the intersectionality of lived experience within a paradigm of bodied-embodied existence and identity, we must remember to challenge and critique all assumptions made about gender within general debates (Shields 301), particularly within childbearing theory and practice. This gendered difference in body and bodily autonomy is fully tied up with the link between maternal identity and the embodied experience of pregnancy. Identity relates to social categories that people associate with themselves (Shields). For the childbearing woman, identity involves a relationship between self and society that changes according to a set of gendered and socially constructed norms, which include a normative view of the woman's behaviours during pregnancy and as a mother. Showing women forceps with no explanation of how they could be used without significant pain and trauma fosters a psychological dependence on the medical world to save the women from their body, which according to dominant discourse is destined to fail.

Stephanie Shields argues that "identity, such as gender or social class, may be experienced as a feature of individual selves, but it also reflects the operation of power relationships among groups that comprise that identity category" (302). These power relations are played out within the embodied experience of motherhood as a uniquely female experience.[1] Expectations of nonfemale parents are different than those whose bodies or identities are female. Although Shields further argues that people are not identified by one single category or descriptor in terms of our identity (304), it is important to remember that for the childbearing woman, biological reproduction becomes the single most important signifier of her identity and social status in the eyes of the wider world. Therefore, a signifier of a woman's status as mother seems to be her ability to survive the loss of autonomy, the violation of her own body, and the loss of dignity and privacy, which is what women, it seems, expect will happen, particularly during their first pregnancies.

In my hypnobirthing classes, couples have said that the frank and detailed explanations I provide about birth, and their rights around birth, have enabled them to feel empowered and to make better choices. The debates and discussions in these classes reinforce what midwifery knowledge and the larger literature have already shown—empowered pregnancy is an embodied one within a paradigm of maternal autonomy.

Pregnancy is well established in the literature as "an embodied and lived experience," which "sets up a range of dichotomies between mind and body, lived and technocratic, subject and object" (Thornham 2). But this divisive debate seems counterproductive when working with women and focusing on empowerment within and through childbearing and motherhood, as I have done for many years as a midwife and midwife teacher. Helen Thornham's research, for example, demonstrates that women's subject position is both "contradictory and negotiated," and their experience is affected by their engagement with pregnancy, childbirth, and technology (2). Technology is viewed as an "ambiguous and anxiety-provoking entity that through its mediations reveals and returns the women to the long-standing tensions and emplaced, embodied subjectivity of maternal identity" (Thornham 2). This research, like so much in this field, emphasizes how women feel little or no sense of control over their pregnancy and birth. I firmly believe that this is one of the primary issues within maternity care and motherhood studies.

My research on midwifery student narratives underpins this fact, and shows that midwives are also subject to the same social forces as women, including forces that place the responsibility for 'healthy' bodies and pregnancies onto women regardless of the other social, societal, and environmental factors which impact on their health. These forces, including paternalistic government guidance and biased, predominantly stereotypical views of gender and women's role in reproduction are enshrined in guidance and publications which continue to undermine women's autonomy because all must be sacrificed on the altar of the perfect baby. Midwives are increasingly limited because of the threat of litigation and professional retribution, which makes them more likely to follow guidelines that do not place the woman as the central controlling figure in the childbirth experience, as suggested by my research on the socialization of midwives through professional education (Einion, "The Socialisation" 190). In 2018, I repeated this earlier study of student midwives' learning journals, following a period of guidance given to these student colleagues on changing the language used to frame professional learning experiences. The journals were used to encourage reflection on professional learning and development each week and to set learning goals for future clinical and academic learning, and to evidence aspects of professional practice to support the students' clinical assessment grading. I carried out a narrative analysis of a small sample of journals that had previously been submitted for assessment.

Initial results demonstrated the discord between the midwife-self and the discourses of the practice area: students either accepted the dominant discourse of medical control or else suffered considerable dissonance between self (including values, beliefs, and ideology) and professional practice. They experienced very real risk of either academic failure or professional censure and litigation. Within these student narratives, there is evidence of students resisting the defensive practice of their mentors and colleagues. At the same time they were creative in writing about this resistance and referred to it very obliquely. Challenging dominant power structures may result in student midwives being denied access to the closed circles of practice colleagues. Left on the margins, these advocates for women's rights feel more vulnerable and more at risk because of their outsider status. They have dared to challenge the status quo, in which patriarchal medicine claims authority over the midwifery profession.

The history of pregnancy, childbearing, and maternal embodiment—the material, personal, and lived experience of childbearing—is tied up with these gendered power relations, which still undermine women's autonomy and agency, and affect maternal subjectivity. Pregnancy and birth, and to a lesser extent mothering, are all biological processes, experienced individually through the body-self, but which are subject to investigation and definition by science and all its co-conspirators—including technology. Thus, science—which neglects many other aspects of female physiology (for example, sexual response or the long-term impact of hormonal birth control)—has made it its business to seize control of pregnancy and childbearing. Many of my clients, for example, are not aware that they can choose where they birth or that they can decline interventions. Women are often unaware of their absolute bodily autonomy during pregnancy and birth. The objectification of the female body by patriarchal institutions remains a key feminist argument (Shildrick), but it is overlooked in many mainstream research studies addressing pregnancy and childbearing, particularly those within the fields of obstetrics and midwifery. It is clear that pregnancy, birth, and motherhood are regulated and controlled by "patriarchal imperatives" (Sutherland et al. 102), but as with so many other constructions of identity and gender, it is very much a performative process (Butler; Neiterman). Pregnancy and childbearing must be performed according to convention, just as midwives must both perform and perpetuate systems of oppression and control.

Expectation and control are manifested through discourse, practice, and lived experience, within which the woman's identity as an individual becomes subsumed into the predefined identity of mother, with the expectation she will conform to the norms of the good mother (Neiterman). In my previous research on childbirth narratives, I discussed how submission is often viewed as not only normative but desirable and that women who resist the control dynamics of healthcare providers are presented as deviant and dangerous (Einion "Resistance and Submission" 179). Women in labour are expected to hand over control of their body and their birth to professionals who know better than them. But no professional, no matter how well educated or experienced, knows a woman's body better than that woman herself. The paternalistic expectation of compliance with dominant discourses around pregnancy and childbearing derives from a long history of science ignoring the embodied knowledge of the women themselves

The debate here hangs on the notion of choice. The question I raise is whether women can exercise informed choice if they cannot access knowledge about the ways society constructs that normalizing discourse. Essentially, no one seems to question medical control of pregnancy and birth because it is deemed a necessary part of the process, which ensures that safety of the mother and baby. This essentialist, reductionist view of childbearing is challenged within midwifery and feminist discourse, research, and debate, but the full empowerment of women in childbearing is no closer to realization than it was in 1993, in the UK, when Changing Childbirth introduced the key principles of choice, continuity, and control as core practices for birth care.

Within this arena, medical surveillance of pregnancy and birth is viewed as the optimal approach. I do not argue against the need to provide all women with access to antenatal care and skilled attendance in labour. But the one-size-fits-all approach to standardizing every aspect of pregnancy and birth completely overlooks individuality, agency, choice, control, and bodily autonomy. Medicine is a vital part of promoting maternal and infant health. But medicine, fully aligned with a technocratic model of health and disease, should not attempt to separate the individual woman from her pregnancy. Medical models of the body present pregnancy as a point of divergence from bodily autonomy. The woman is no longer an individual whose rights and choices are her own. Suddenly, she is a mother, and she is expected to set aside her individuality and identity as she ascends to the throne of motherhood and submits to all forms of surveillance and control deemed culturally appropriate.

Women who live and birth within a Western medical paradigm have grown to view medically managed birth as the norm (Kennedy et al.)—a view perpetuated and reinforced by media portrayals of birth and childbearing as risky, frightening, and fraught with tension (Einion "Resistance and Submission" 178). Yet women often remain unaware of the potential complications of the medical interventions purported to make their birth safer. For example, in my hypnobirthing classes, I spend as much time discussing women's various upcoming birth choices as I do developing their skills in hypnotic relaxation. They are otherwise afforded limited information about routine medical interventions—such as vaginal examinations, epidural anesthesia, opiates offered for pain management, or the oxytocic drugs used to expedite the delivery of the placenta. They often do not know the side effects of these interventions or their long-term impact on their wellbeing or their infants'.

Thus, in Western culture, the female body remains defined as inherently problematic (Jeffreys 5), and this conceptualization is powerfully constructed through and by language. It is important here to draw the distinction between bodies as cultural products rather than as collections of biological structures and processes (Gatens 35). A challenge to the medical hegemonic surveillance of the pregnant body cannot be divorced from the ways in which women are perceived and represented by the media, and I include in this not just the broadcast media and populist publications, which the lay person is exposed to, but the other media that fuel the machine of medical and healthcare practice—the research literature. The paradigms defining the nature of healthcare practice are fully grounded in a patriarchal discourse and model, which affords power only to those who adhere to this scientific norm.

Science does not allow for women to be recognized as women within their social context; it reduces them to bodies, parts of bodies, and statistics. Through this dominance, the medical establishment, fully supported by governments and politicians, limits the knowledge available to women (and men) and even limits the forms in which that knowledge may be disseminated. In setting the standards for what it will accept as evidence for healthcare practice, the medical establishment acts as another cultural force—it sets the expectations for an entire society and refuses to acknowledge the value of any other viewpoint. It accepts only certain types of research as evidence; studies in which childbearing women's voices are solicited, sourced, and represented are not accepted as evidence for practice. The woman's experience is viewed as of lesser importance in the face of medicine, despite the thousands of years of bodily knowing and biological evolution she carries within her. Challenging this view is further complicated by the emergence of more and more investigation into the science of epigenetics, which focuses on the impact of maternal behaviours on the infant genome and which increases the weight of science's critical gaze (Meloni).

It is understandable that women adhere to a socially accepted worldview that their pregnancy needs surveillance. The first message women receive about their pregnancy is that something could go wrong; therefore, medicine must constantly monitor them. Women bear the weight of this worldview, yet it is essentially opposed to the simple biological facts of pregnancy and childbearing. Women's bodies are made to bear and birth children, but this message is not what women hear when they access information from healthcare profess-ionals and the media. These messages fail to reinforce key dimensions of childbearing: bodily and personal autonomy and choice, and the body's innate ability to birth, given the right conditions.

Bodily and personal autonomy have been the subject of endless debate within midwifery. Despite the rhetoric of midwifery (particularly in the UK) purporting to provide women-centred care, women's autonomy is not generally respected once women enter the healthcare arena. The status of healthcare providers as experts creates a hierarchy in which the woman occupies a lower position supposedly because of her lack of expertise. Again, my experiences with women completely reinforce this viewpoint, particularly women having their first babies. They enter my classes hoping to find a way to be in control and to cope with the birth experience, yet they do not have the belief in their own ability to birth. Instead, they enter a strange environment, and let everyone else tell them what is best for them and their bodies and their babies. Their lack of knowledge is staggering, and ultimately, disempowering. The medical narrative dominates all other narratives, including our own self-story As Arthur Frank argues, "the obligation of seeking medical care [becomes] a narrative surrender" (6). Not all women, however, simply relinquish control once they become pregnant and seek healthcare. Women negotiate their way through the relationship by managing their personal and bodily autonomy in different ways (Westfall and Benoit).

Yet women do seek medical surveillance because of their sense of destabilization during pregnancy. Pregnancy involves significant physiological change—changes in hormones changes, in body size and shape, in cardiovascular function, in the digestive system, and in mood—such that the experience of pregnancy anchors the woman in her physical reality. Medical control of pregnancy knowledge—including the simple act of having someone else (i.e., a doctor) confirm the pregnancy's reality and viability—competes with the woman's bodily knowledge of pregnancy. Pregnancy is not real until it is confirmed by the establishment. It is not safe until the woman has undergone a dating scan to confirm her due date and an anomaly scan to check for viability. The woman's own bodily knowledge of her pregnancy, and even her date of conception, is disregarded. A woman may know the exact days in which she was ovulating, and the exact date on which she had exposure to sperm, and the exact date of the first day of her last menstrual period, but all this information is disregarded because it has not come from a doctor.

In my first pregnancy, I knew I was pregnant from the day I conceived. As I fell asleep the evening after a day on the beach, where we swam in the sea and made love on a headland, I dreamed of conception. I dreamed of darkness, and a little light joining a bigger light. I woke up and knew I was pregnant. In my second pregnancy, I suspected I was pregnant and carried out several home pregnancy tests over a period of two weeks. My colleagues were constantly telling me I looked pregnant (yes, midwives are that good), and I knew instinctively that I was. But the tests were all negative. Therefore, I kept telling myself I was not pregnant, just stressed. I knew however that I had conceived during my three days off work at Christmas. My son was born on 24 September, nine months after the conception that was not initially confirmed by scientific testing. This story echoes ones clients often tell me about their own experience of conception and the fact that it is not real until medically confirmed. Thus, the woman's authority over self is disregarded in pregnancy, which feeds the notion that the pregnancy is not hers. She has become a vessel and is responsible to the wider world for the life that she carries, which contravenes any notion of individual rights.

Social institutions have too much power over the individual rights of childbearing women; they position woman as subordinate not only to social rules but to the needs, wellbeing, and existence of her child. The tendency toward detailed interrogation of pregnancy, both through human and through technological means, continues to be supported by science.

Women are not machines. Much of maternity care in the Western world is already provided as a kind of conveyor belt of assessment, referral, treatment, and transfer from one clinical area to another. Midwives have little scope to practice autonomously or to observe the impact of this kind of care on students, colleagues, and clients. By increasing the monitoring and management of pregnancy and birth, medicine grows stronger and limits women's choices. The factors limiting these rights often have little to do with clinical need but with the institutions within which birth takes place. At the time of writing, the UK Nursing and Midwifery council have published an edict saying that the indemnity insurance provided by Independent Midwives UK is no longer sufficient for independent midwives to provide intrapartum care. This means that women have no choice. Either they must access NHS services, and all their attendant problems, or they must choose to birth without a midwife.

The relationship between power, control, and the embodiment of motherhood continues to be challenged by mothers and midwives alike. Yet Wendy Savage attests the following:

> Despite the rhetoric about "choice" for women in childbirth, and "openness and transparency" in governance, there is still a lot to do if women are to be able to give birth in the way they wish to and if all those involved in health care are to be truly accountable to the wider society they serve.... The issue of birth and power is one which arouses strong emotions, because birth is a profoundly moving experience for all those who participate in the drama, whether as the person who should be the central point of the whole event, the woman, or the person who should be in a supporting role, the midwife or doctor. (3)

The very language used here to describe the expected dynamic of birth also obliquely refers to the actuality of the birth experience. Savage says "should" because regardless of the current rhetoric, or the professional discourse of midwifery, women are not the central focus of birth within a Western medicalized paradigm. Their survival, as well as the infants', is the focus.

As Katz Rothman suggests, the "first thing to remember is that obstetrics is a surgical specialty. The management of childbirth within hospitals is essentially the same as the management of any other surgical event" (163). Thus, women are not viewed as people but as biological machines. Women are still coerced during decision-making processes: if they do not adhere to medical instructions, then they are putting their baby at risk. The absolutism of these assertions is, frankly, wrong. Nothing guarantees that the infant will be well. Pregnancy and birth are times of uncertainty. But women are set up to expect that if they submit to the birth surveillance, the outcome will be positive. At the same time, women also place their trust, and a large degree of control over their person, into the hands of someone else because that person knows more about obstetrics. It is understandable that a woman seeks reassurance during pregnancy and childbearing, an experience which has always been fearful and emotionally laden.

The surveillance and consequent intervention that women not only accept but actively seek out does not guarantee better outcomes, and some practices, such as ultrasound scanning and induction of labour, have been established as standard practice without robust evidence of their contribution to positive outcomes (Savage 344). Even the term "positive outcomes" can be questioned because what this means for the institutions of obstetrics and of society may not match with the real lived experience of women bearing children.

What has this to do with maternal embodiment? In *Bodies that Matter,* Judith Butler states that "what constitutes the fixity of the body, its contours, its movements, will be fully material, but materiality will be rethought as the effect of power, as power's most productive effect" (130). She further states that when the nature of gender as a social construct and the nature of normativity according to gender are understood, then "the materiality of the body will not be thinkable apart from the materialization of that regulatory norm" (130). For the childbearing woman, her bodily experience is regulated by culturally assigned norms of childbearing—such as weight and shape (espoused in the fundamentally and famously flawed body mass index calculation), weight gain, age, and risk status, where risk is a constructed concept based on medical parameters of normal vs abnormal.

Who gave the healthcare profession the power to define what is normal? As Grantly Dick-Read so eloquently put it, when did the interloper creep in? Butler's concept of symbolic legitimacy is key here. A patriarchal institution has defined the symbolic legitimacy of the embodied subject within a defined set of parameters that constitute normal or low risk. But this is only an extension of the wider social construct of women's embodiment of this form of compulsory femaleness, which condemns them to a life of childbearing to gain social legitimacy, as long as they do so within strictly defined parameters. Thus, this system not only requires women to be mothers—viewing the choice not to bear children at best as selfish and at worst as immoral—but also requires them to become mothers in socially acceptable ways. This requirement is achieved through a baseless and essentially falsified transaction: if you behave as we want you to, you and your baby will survive. Yet this transaction also rests on thee falsehood that childbirth is inevitably both fearful and painful and that the maternal body in its natural and uninterrupted state is doomed to fail. This is not the case, as Sarah Buckley shows in her report on the hormonal physiology of childbearing. It is the interruptions to that physiology, of professionals entering the room unnecessarily, or leaving birth room doors open, or placing time limits on labour, for example, that precipitate the problems in many cases.

No one can guarantee a positive outcome for pregnancy and childbearing. The lack of agency in women's accounts of childbearing, as well as their lack of dignity and autonomy, shows that maternal embodiment during this period must involve submission of their self (or, in dualistic terms, their body) to another. The woman sacrifices herself (and her body) for her children. This sacrifice is not only acceptable in our current social context but desirable, yet it is paradoxically also seen as problematic because being pregnant deviates from the dominant cultural norms of body slenderness. Women's bodies matter, to echo Judith Butler's use of the term, only to those who erroneously perceive they have some ownership of that body. The loss of bodily autonomy relates to the idea that the fetus is more important than its mother, and has its own rights. Through submission to external control, the woman can guarantee the child's survival and wellbeing. This is a falsehood.

Many years ago, I wrote a paper for a conference examining the status of the fetus in law and in practice. I was motivated by my personal experience of a discourse I can only call "the cult of the fetus," which prioritizes the wellbeing of the fetus and labels women who fight for control of their childbearing and their bodies as selfish. I came into midwifery believing that all women had the right to choose how they bear and birth children. Twenty-one years later, I still believe this is the case, but women themselves do not know how much their bodily autonomy is being eroded. I have lost count of the midwives who have talked about a woman who was induced for being past her due date and the baby was born looking as if it was a much earlier gestation than had been supposed. I have lost count of the women who speak of leaving their dignity at the door when they go into hospital to birth. Women feel they are unimportant. They feel that their bodily existence is unimportant and belongs to someone else. In no other area of social or personal life are individuals relegated to such a subordinate position without question or challenge. In no other area of social life are people's bodily autonomy transgressed by others without full knowledge and understanding of what is to be done.

As I write, I am reviewing the recent World Health Organization guideline on care during birth, which advocates against anticipatory intervention in the natural bodily processes of birth, and for a culture of respectful care. The need to stress respect in this guideline indicates there is a deficit in many current practices. Dick-Read discusses this lack of respect in his book, which was first published in the middle of the twentieth century. Midwives continue to use his work as the basis of activities and support approaches that foster the physiological experience of birth without separating it from the woman who is undergoing that experience. His method of childbirth preparation and management uses hypnotic techniques and education to empower women to both feel in control of the birth experience and also to connect on a deep level to the biological processes taking place within her: "It is a method which enables women to have their children by physiological principles and mechanism with which the healthy human female is equipped for that purpose ... designed to protect women from the appalling dangers of ignorance. This not only applies to mothers but to those who look after them from conception to the end of the puerperium" (153).

His book is titled *Childbirth without Fear,* and it has taken me over twenty years as a midwife to come to a deep understanding of the scope and meaning of that title. For much of my career, I believed that this title referred to removing women's fear of childbearing. But I also believe that it relates to removing the fear of childbirth from the medical profession, midwifery, society and Western culture. We fear what we cannot control. We are taught to believe that our bodies are not ours to control and that childbearing is something in which we relinquish control. As Nancy Stoller Shaw states, "This does not mean that the woman becomes unimportant, only that her body, or more specifically, the birth canal and its contents, and the almost born baby are the only things the doctor is really interested in" (qtd. in Katz Rothman 165). The embodied fetus becomes the primary focus of the experience, and women who make their own choices are viewed as selfish. Women are not supposed to be selfish in our culture; they are supposed to be long-suffering and self-sacrificing. Pregnancy is not viewed as a life event in which a mother has a full and meaningful experience. It is simply what must be endured to give her the reward of a baby. Instead of embracing the experience, many women resist and fight what is entirely physiologically natural. They fight the increase in body fat, which occurs in order to feed their child during pregnancy and after birth. They fight the increase in body size, and set goals to lose their baby weight. Pregnancy is a time when mothers begin that process of becoming a mother, one which will be defined and refined throughout their life course. But none of this is valued in the Western paradigm. The baby takes precedence. Without it, the pregnancy becomes meaningless. Pregnancy is defined as purposeful. If a woman becomes pregnant, but fails to produce a live child, she is deemed to have failed. The pregnancy was a waste of time.

I speak from personal experience as well as from many years of professional experience and knowledge. When I was twenty years old, I became pregnant for the first time. I loved it. I embraced the whole experience. I wondered and marvelled at the changes in my body. I fully believed in its ability to carry the mysterious new person living inside me. I loved the feel of him moving, the increase in sensation in various parts of my skin, the appearance of colostrum, and the change in body shape. I loved being pregnant. I had never planned to have children. I had not spent my childhood and adolescence dreaming of marriage and baby names and of decorating the nursery. Far from it. I was convinced, right up until the moment I conceived, that I would be happier without children. I had no urge to reproduce or to become a mother. But when this embodied state of motherhood became my reality, I loved it.

I was labelled as deviant by mainstream society because of my lifestyle at the time, and I had little or no knowledge of how the medical system worked or what their expectations of me were. I was shocked when the midwife in the clinic weighed me and made negative comments about being overweight. I was invited to antenatal classes, but these were difficult to attend, as they were far away and the bus was expensive. I was not told to make appointments at the local antenatal clinic. I was labelled a non-attender, and, therefore, irresponsible. I was completely unaware of their labelling of me.

Yet I was fully in love with pregnancy and with understanding the mystery and power that came with my transition to motherhood. It was a deeply spiritual experience. I believed so strongly in the absolute ability of my body to bear a child that I was not worried about the birth, but I was concerned about having the kind of birth I wanted. And I did, up until the last two hours when I was deemed to need "speeding up" and medicine took over. Even afterward, I still felt this strong connection to myself, my spirit, and this new being born during that process—my mother identity.

Then the baby died.

Suddenly none of what happened mattered to anyone else. In the eyes of society, I was not a mother. Without the product of that experience to validate my identity, I was not seen as a mother, and my experience could not be shared. The profound nature of my grief was exacerbated by the sudden transition to nonmother. I had lost not only the child I loved but a huge part of myself. And no one cared. Most people simply said, "well, you can have another one," as if all that mattered was the physical reality of a child, any child, to prove my status as mother. I still felt empowered by the experience of childbearing; I felt I had gained wisdom, insight, and a deeper and wider view of the world. During the birth, I had my moment of epiphany: I understood midwifery to be my calling. It was a life-changing event, and despite experiencing the greatest sadness I have ever known—an almost bottomless well of emotional agony that will never fully leave me—I also felt stronger and more capable and fulfilled because it was a watershed moment that cast everything into perspective. Talking about the experience in anything but negative terms, though, made people uncomfortable, so I learned to keep it to myself. It was seen as selfish to say that it was a life-enhancing experience. Nothing else I attached to the experience mattered because I didn't have a baby to prove my social worth. To be empowered by losing a child runs counter to every discourse within obstetrics. Refusing to believe that I had failed as a mother is an act of resistance, of both the prevailing narrative and the constructions of punishment that I 'should' experience for my deviance in not submitting to the surveillance of my pregnancy in the prescribed manner.

Pregnancy and birth have always been socially constructed because of a dynamic interaction between the individual and the social context. Dominant ideals, ideologies, and myths surrounding childbearing are perpetuated through the control of information and knowledge. This control of information around women's health, empowerment, and childbearing capacity has been the business of patriarchal institutions throughout history, and it continues to be perpetuated by Western healthcare systems. Had I had then the knowledge I have now, things might have been different. And I fully believe that every single woman should be educated to the same level as any midwife so that they can retain control over their lives and have the tools with which to build a fortress of personal and bodily autonomy that cannot be breached.

There is a danger, of course, inherent in my own position as academic, midwife, and author of this chapter because I write from a position of power and assert my opinion as valid and weighty. Maybe some women will argue that ignorance is bliss and that they prefer to hand over power, responsibility, and control to knowledgeable professionals. Certainly, I have encountered many such women in my professional and personal life. Have I any right to say that their position is wrong? Have I any right to assert that all women should question everything that they know or understand about their persons? Have I any right to argue that their desire for aspects of their self to be monitored, judged, evaluated, and directed by an external agency, is in fact wrong? Perhaps not.

It is, however, a fundamental point. Despite my greater knowledge, I am not in possession of all the facts, but then again, no one is. I cannot know why Mrs. X is so frightened of having an epidural, or why Miss Y wants to listen to whale song during her birth. But if Miss Y wants a whale song, then she should have the whale song, regardless of whether she births in a yurt under a tree in a far-flung field or in a high-tech operating theatre with surgeons assisting her. She should retain that sense of control while accessing her safety net of skilled midwives and obstetricians who are there for her and her baby and are a vital part of her support team. More than once I have viewed obstetricians—professionals whom I admire and deeply respect, whose input and skills I value very highly—fail to recognize their own assumption of superiority. For example, when I worked as a delivery suite midwife, I frequently acted as the scrub midwife for Caesarean sections. There was a CD player in each theatre. With one client, who was having a planned Caesarean, I checked what music she wanted and loaded it in the player. I tried to create a positive and calm environment to help my client to relax. I told her "just focus on your music, but if you want us to explain exactly what we are doing, we can do that too."

Upon entering in his gown, mask, and gloves, the surgeon, instead of greeting my conscious client, simply said, "Well, you can turn that rubbish off right now. I want Genesis on." I thought he would understand perfectly when I explained the importance of the music. His response, however, was one of confusion: "But this is *my* theatre."

I have for many years viewed midwives as gatekeepers, acting as a portal between woman and institution, and as a guardian to women's autonomy. The ideology of midwifery is akin to that of feminism: an inherited and deliberately constructed conceptual field in which women are placed at the primacy of every discourse. In practice, midwives who work within the regulatory landscape of the UK are as oppressed as the women they serve because they are limited in their ability to protect and promote that autonomy. Surveillance of pregnancy and birth as defined by our institutional norms is a form of control, and both professional and institutional systems feed into the mechanism of clinical governance—a quality assurance model with the prime goal of reducing the cost of litigation. Midwives are ultimately subject to this clinical governance and to professional controls, which limit their power to support women in their choices.

Maternal surveillance, which is the primary role of the midwife in the Western paradigm, views the woman's body, and therefore, the woman herself, as nothing more than a means of production, set about with a panoply of risks, couched in terms of safety and wellbeing. Pregnancy is, thus, something to be monitored and controlled, regardless of the fact that this a woman's personal life experience. Once a woman becomes a mother, she embodies a social reality that appears to be owned by the institutions of society. And that ownership requires women to submit to surveillance without questioning its purpose and its potential outcomes, which is fuelled by a history of mothers being both worshipped and admired yet ultimately blamed for all the ills of society and for failing to be a 'good enough' mother (Ladd-Taylor). I can only conclude, based on years of experience within this domain, that to carry a baby is to carry the weight of expectation of society and to find your pregnancy co-opted and owned by others. Maternal surveillance makes the childbearing body the property of the state, and few people seem disturbed by this reality.

Yet I regularly see women and their partners becoming empowered through acquiring knowledge, through using of positive birth language, and through seeing a small number of midwives advocating for women's absolute bodily autonomy and individual rights. In the anonymous evaluations of my hypnobirthing classes, women state they feel confident in their ability to birth at the end of the classes, even if they did not feel confident prior to the classes. The comments show that understanding the level of choice and control one has during birth is an important part of parents exercising their autonomy.

From this knowledge, there is only one way forward. Women must resist. Midwives and doctors must resist. In order to remove the barriers to women experiencing an empowered birth we must all stand up and advocate for women's autonomy and their absolute right to self-determination. We must educate and support women to gain the knowledge and understanding that will afford them the power to change the way our social institutions categorizes them. We must become aware of the purpose of surveillance medicine when applied to the female body and of the danger of using language that divorces bodily reality from personhood. We must promote a form of equality that both affords women access to medical intervention and enables them to understand the limitations of science and medicine. And we must deconstruct the opinions that label women as mere vessels and work to rewrite the birth script in a language that celebrates the power and beauty of the birthing body. Childbearing is wonderful, and wonderfully challenging. Those of us called to serve childbearing women should see ourselves in that way, as servants to the mother, without whom there is no family, there is no society, and there is no future.

The birthing woman breathes; her eyes are half-closed. One hand is on the turgid mound of the womb, taut with the power of the birthing surge. Caught up in the changes, in the wavelike movements of the womb muscle, she breathes deeply, settles into the sensations, and rides the waves, trough to crest and back again, powerfully in control. She is fully engaged with her birthing. She knows that she is surrounded by calm and that there are people with skills to assist her available should she need them. She trusts, fully, in her body, in her birth partner, in her love for her baby, and in her transition to parenthood. She accepts the power and intensity of the birthing sensations. She chooses to birth in the way she wants to.

Endnote

1 I do not exclude trans or genderqueer persons with wombs, but their experience of childbearing is uniquely different from the cisgender female experience, which is the focus of this chapter. To do justice to the experience of trans* or genderqueer persons bearing children would require far more consideration and focus than is possible in the scope of this discussion.

Works Cited

Bordo, Susan. *Unbearable Weight: Feminism, Western Culture and the Body.* University of California Press, 2003.

Buckley, Sarah J. *Hormonal Physiology of Childbearing: Evidence and Implications for Women, Babies, and Maternity Care.* Childbirth Connection Programs, National Partnership for Women & Families, January 2015.

Butler, Judith. *Bodies That Matter: On the Discursive Limits of the "Sex.* Routledge, 1993.

Carter, Shannon K. "Beyond Control: Body and Self in Women's Childbearing Narratives." *Sociology of Health and Illness,* vol. 32, no. 7, 2010, pp. 993-1009.

Dick-Read, G. *Childbirth Without Fear.* Pinter and Martin 2013
Einion, Alys. "The Socialisation of Student Midwives: Rewriting the Landscape." *The Social Context of Birth,* edited by Caroline Squire, CRC Press, 2017, pp. 181-92.

Einion, Alys. "Resistance and Submission: A Critique of Representations of Birth." *Natal Signs: Cultural Representations of Pregnancy, Birth and Parenting*, edited by Nadya Burton. Demeter Press, 2015, pp. 172-93.

Frank, Arthur. *The Wounded Storyteller: Body, Illness and Ethics.* Chicago University Press, 1995.

Gatens, Moira. *Imaginary bodies: Ethics, Power and Corporeality.* Routledge, 2013.

Jeffreys, Sheila. Beauty and *Misogyny: harmful cultural practices in the West.* Routledge, 2005.

Kennedy, Holly P., et al. "Top-Selling Childbirth Advice Books: A Discourse Analysis." *Birth*, vol. 36, 2009, pp.318-324.

Ladd-Taylor, Molly. "Mother-Worship/Mother-Blame." *Maternal Theory: Essential Readings*, edited by Andrea O'Reilly, Demeter, 2007, pp. 660-67.

Meloni, Maurizion. "Epigenetics for the Social Sciences: Justice, Embodiment, and Inheritance in the Postgenomic Age." *New Genetics and Society*, vol. 34, no. 2, 2015, pp. 125-51.

Neiterman, Elena. "Doing Pregnancy: Pregnant Embodiment as Performance." *Women's Studies International Forum*, vol. 35, 2012, 373-83.

Rothman, Barbara Katz. *Recreating Motherhood.* Rutgers University Press, 2000.

Savage, Wendy. *Birth and Power: A Savage Enquiry Revisited.* Middlesex University Press, 2007.

Shields, Stephanie A. "Gender: An Intersectionality Perspective." *Sex Roles*, vol. 59, 2008, pp. 301-11.

Shildrick, Margit. *Leaky Bodies and Boundaries: Feminism, Postmodernism and (Bio) Ethics.* Routledge, 1997.

Sutherland, Olga, et al. "Digital Actualizations of Gender and Embodiment: Microanalysis of Onine Pregnancy Discourse." *Women's Studies International Forum*, vol. 47, 2014, pp. 102-14.

Thornham, Helen. "Irreconcilability in the Digital: Gender, Technological Imaginings and Maternal Subjectivity." *Feminist Review*, vol. 110, 2015, pp. 1-17.

Westfall, Rachel, and Ceclia Benoit. "Interpreting Compliance and Resistance to Medical Dominance in Women's Accounts of their Pregancies." *Sociological Research Online*, vol. 13, no. 3-4, 2008, p.4.

Chapter Two

Dangerous Bodies: Imagining, Monitoring, and Managing Fatness during Pregnancy

Megan Davidson and Sarah Lewin

In a New York Times article titled Pregnant, Obese ... and in Danger, obstetrician Claire Putman argues that the health of the nation rests upon the shoulders of fat people. "Obesity in mothers," she writes, "is strongly linked to their own compromised health, and to that of their unborn babies and our nation at large." Doctors bombard pregnant people with the message that fat bodies are dangerous, which is used to authorize extensive medical management. Fat[1] parents are shamed for endangering themselves, their future child, and even the nation with a list of complications that continues to grow: diabetes, preeclampsia, hypertension, infection, birth loss, big babies, and birth defects, among others. Putnam notes that she sees a growing number of "super obese" patients and finds it "frightening to think that this might become normal." Sentiments such as Putnam's highlight the hysteria around the growing weight of Americans and the fear of fat bodies. Deeply rooted aggression toward large-bodied pregnant people, masked in concerns around health, drives a moralizing narrative about which bodies should reproduce and parent—and which should not.

Jonathan Metzl writes in his 2010 book *Against Health*: "'Health' is a term replete with value judgments, hierarchies, and blind assumptions that speak as much about power and privilege as they do about well-being. Health is a desired state, but it is also a prescribed state and an ideological position" (1-2). Metzl defends the "against health" position of the authors and explains that they are, like us, not denying the importance of medicine or science and not suggesting we stop researching and innovating. Rather, as Richard Klein writes, "To be against health ... is to be critical of the myths and lies concerning our health that are circulated by the media and paid for by large industries. It is to demystify their hidden moralizing and their political agenda, exposing what we might properly call the current ideology of health" (16-17). This concept of health overwhelms us. Endless images and messages are deployed to remind us that it is our obligation to pursue thinness. Kathleen LeBesco, in her essay "Fat Panic and the New Morality," uses the phrase "moral panic" to describe the hostility and outrage directed at fat people (73). She writes, "our insistence on turning efforts to achieve good health into a greater moral enterprise means that health also becomes a sharp political stick in which much harm is ultimately done" (78). This moral panic around diet, body size, and fatness—our ideology of health—is the health we are also against.

All people, regardless of their size, deserve compassionate, non-judgmental care, and access to evidence-based information so that they can make the best decisions for themselves. Emily Oster, economist and author of the bestselling pregnancy book *Expecting Better*, writes that prenatal care is often approached as "one long list of rules"; parents-to-be are treated like "a child again" rather than being meaningfully engaged in thoughtful decision making (xv). During one of the more important and meaningful times in most people's lives, "we are often not given the opportunity to think critically about the decisions we make. Instead we are expected to follow a largely arbitrary script without question" (Oster xxii).

For fat pregnant people this 'largely arbitrary script' is one steeped in current public health dialogues that have demonized fatness, naturalized thinness, and removed the possibility of a healthy fat body. With a "war on obesity" being waged, healthy fat bodies are clinically and culturally incomprehensible: there is no such thing as benign fatness (Bacon; Campos et al.; LeBesco; Wann). Fatphobia affects all people, but women uniquely navigate unrealistic standards dictating how, and in what kind of body, femaleness (and motherhood) can be performed. Embedded in understandings of woman and mother is a raced and classed expectation of body maintenance, which has become the symbol for health, purity, success, and virtuosity. Furthermore, modern-day healthisms place the responsibility of being in good health on the individual, distracting from larger determinants of health such as race and socioeconomic status. Fat pregnant people must navigate the gauntlet of normal pregnancy-induced concerns and pressures on parents while their decision to reproduce is at best seen as suspect and at worst as a selfish endangering of their future child.

In the U.S. cultural imagination, fatness remains rigidly coded as dangerous, risky, undesirable, and immoral—the antithesis of what a mother should be. Scientific claims of difference rooted in the body are used to solidify power claims and make our differences appear to be "natural, inevitable, even god-given" (Yanagisako and Delaney 1). In this essay, we unpack scientific claims about obesity, and challenge the belief that fatness is always dangerous. The monitoring and management of so-called risky bodies throughout pregnancy do not make people safer or healthier but rather helps to naturalize, authorize, and (re) produce narratives of fat as unhealthy and immoral. We conclude our essay by considering alternative approaches to prenatal care and identifying sites of resistance in which pregnant people birth healthy babies and reclaim their dangerous maternal bodies.

Dangerous Bodies

Pregnant people are watched closely by onlookers, and their bodies are open to public judgment. They are disciplined, beginning in the early stages of pregnancy, to understand their weight and their child's weight as an essential expression of parental success. Popular culture, film, and television, friends and family, and health professionals all remind pregnant people of the obligation to remain thin and fit, even while gestating. Notions of irrational food cravings—indulgently "eating for two"—foster stereotypes of pregnant people needing to discipline unruly and illicit desires in direct conflict with the wellbeing of their baby. Fetishizations of the slender pregnant body as well as an emphasis on a quick return to a fit body postpartum are perpetually featured in magazines. Pregnant people of all sizes experience body shaming and weight policing in the form of cultural pressure and medical staff armed with strict weight-monitoring guidelines (IOM). Success and failure are made numerical on the scale.

Being pregnant in a sizeist culture presents unique challenges to all people adjusting to their growing and changing bodies. These challenges are amplified for fat people, who must navigate multiple layers of complications within reproductive care: first, in access to fertility treatments; next, in prenatal obstetrical treatment; and finally, in the medical management of birth. There is an abundance of data linking obesity to complications; given these "known adverse consequences" (Leddy et al.), fat people seeking fertility treatments are routinely advised that they cannot receive reproductive help at their size. Many fertility centres have body mass index (BMI) requirements, which effectively determines who is fit for parenthood and who is not. In order to achieve acceptable BMI levels, people might be advised to lose enormous amounts of weight—sometimes more than half their body weight—before they can access fertility treatments routinely made available to thinner people, even those with more significant fertility or health problems.

Although weight gain during pregnancy is typically a sign of good health, American anxieties around body size contribute to close weight and food surveillance during pregnancy.[2] Standard care includes routine weigh-ins, prescriptions for low-fat or low-carb diets, a lengthy list of restricted foods, and hospital policies that routinely forbid eating during labour. Fat people—even those who are healthy and for whom all tests indicate no problems—are routinely subjected to increased monitoring. Meaghan Leddy and colleagues suggest that because of the documented risks associated with obesity, routine prenatal care for fat people needs to be adjusted (174). This adjustment is done through increased prenatal appointments and testing, including repeated screenings for gestational diabetes, and through extensive warnings about the risks associated with their weight. Furthermore, many fat pregnant people are advised to lose weight. Since dieting in pregnancy is not advised, this weight loss should not be the result of dieting.

These types of monitoring and prescriptions for limited weight gain (and even weight loss) are the standard of care for fat prenatal patients in the U.S. today. These medical care practices must be seen as "deeply cultural acts" than "cannot be divorced from the cultural and individual contexts in which the care is delivered," as Megan McCullough writes (218). This standard care should not be confused for evidence-based care: "many elements of routine prenatal care are based on tradition and lack a firm evidence base" (Zolotor and Carlough 199). McCullough reminds us that "the body is both a reflection and construction of a culture's values and beliefs" (218). In pregnancy, cultural values and beliefs about healthy and dangerous bodies have outweighed actual data or best practices.

Pregnant people of all sizes are frequently chastised for their weight gain by care providers. They are told that they are gaining too much or that their baby is growing too large. Often this is followed by unfounded criticism masquerading as food advice—"Eat more carrots," "No more cookies," "Only low fat dairy for you," "Cut out the carbs." If they are among the pregnant people who face severe nausea and chronic vomiting, many fat people are told to welcome this as a way to limit weight gain, instead of being given sympathy and medication to help. Fat people face relentless commentary from care providers who tell them that their bodies are dangerous and their babies are at risk.

There are concerning rates of interventions and Caesarean birth across this country—at numbers that make pregnancy less, not more, safe. Fat pregnant people are particularly vulnerable to these unnecessary interventions; they are scheduled for inductions and Caesarean births more often, and they suffer higher numbers of postpartum complications. Assumptions about their pregnancies and labour based on body size often override clinical data. For example, "soft tissue dystocia"—also referred to as the "fat vagina" theory—is the belief that large people have more internal fat stores in their pelvis and birth canal, which complicate vaginal birth (Viraday, "Fat Vagina"). Despite research showing that fat deposits inside the vagina are clinically insignificant, doctors continue to cite soft tissue dystocia as a reason for concern and interventions—affirming narratives of fat bodies as disgusting and flawed.

Routine prenatal care is negatively affected by the understanding of fat bodies as risky and on the verge of illness. Healthy weight gain is incongruent with the "current ideology of health" (Klein 17), and this permeates the experience of pregnancy and prenatal care. Pregnant people must make sense of the conflicting messages they receive daily, including from doctors. Discourse around fatness reflects and shapes narratives of modern parenthood, as well as naturalizes notions of who is fit for parenting and who is not. The monitoring and management of risky patients in pregnancy are not currently making us safer or healthier; rather, they (re)produce narratives of fat as unhealthy and immoral.

Dangerous Data

The history of medicine is filled with examples of erroneous conclusions drawn from bad methodology, which assumes that correlation equals causation. For example, medical researchers Graham Quinn and colleagues found a "strong association" between nearsightedness (myopia) and night-time ambient light exposure in the first two years of life, which led researchers to warn against nightlights in baby's rooms. Subsequent studies failed to prove a causal relationship though (see Guggenheim et al.; Gwiazda et al.; Saw et al.; Zadnick et al.), likely because parents who used nightlights were themselves nearsighted, a heritable trait passed to their children. Similarly, initial support for hormone replacement therapy (HRT) during menopause, as a means to reduce coronary heart disease (CHD), was later discovered to be bad advice because HRT actually put women at greater risk for CHD (Lawlor et al.). As both of these examples demonstrate, the questions we ask, the assumptions we make, and the conclusions we draw from medical data matter enormously and they are often found to be partial, imperfect, or completely wrong.

In her analysis of the unproblematized cultural metaphors that structure our understandings of biological phenomena ("The Egg" 501), the anthropologist Emily Martin reminds us that "it is easier to see how scientific ideas from the past, ideas that now seem wrong or too simple, might have been affected by cultural ideas of an earlier time" (*The Woman* 27). Given the ubiquitous sizeism and fatphobia in contemporary Western culture, and the moral panic around ideologues of health, it is no wonder there is an abundance of scientific inquiry into obesity and the dangers and disease of the fat body. In Western culture, McCullough writes, "obesity is read as a body in distress" (226). Anthropologist Anna Tsing has argued that "cultural agendas create the frameworks and technologies in which observers find natural difference where they need to see it" (114). This is evident in how obesity in pregnancy is being studied and produced as a site of danger.

Currently, the dangers linked to obesity in pregnancy and birth include increased risk of developing gestational diabetes, preeclampsia, and hypertension; greater likelihood of urinary tract infections and postpartum infections; increased risk that pregnancy will continue beyond the expected due date (as well as an increased risk of preterm birth); greater likelihood of induction; greater risk of complications with pain medications such as epidurals; and increased likelihood of both elective and emergency Caesarean birth (alongside decreased likelihood of a successful vaginal birth after a Cesarean birth). Additionally, higher BMI is considered to increase the risk of miscarriage, the risk of delivering an infant significantly larger than average (macrosomia), the risk of the baby developing heart disease or diabetes as an adult, and even (to a slight degree) the risk of having birth defects, such as neural tube defects, as well as having a stillbirth (COG; Buschur and Kim 6, Chu et al.; Leddy et al.; Mayo Clinic). This list continues to grow with new studies routinely linking weight with various fertility, pregnancy, postpartum, and childhood health complications.[3] The message is not subtle—it is dangerous for fat people to have babies.

Care providers treating fat pregnant people often cite alarming statistics: the stillbirth rate is three times higher for fat people; their preeclampsia rate is four times higher; fat people have a 50 percent chance of having a Caesarean birth as well as have an increased risk of preterm birth; and fat people three times as likely to develop gestational diabetes. Furthermore, fat pregnant people might be counselled that their babies are 3.5 times as likely to have neural tube defects and are twice as likely to have congenital heart disease. Being a pregnant person facing this list of risks and complications, while also trying to navigate the greater cultural stigma about body size, can be overwhelming. It is easy to believe that your body is dangerous under these conditions.

Yet the medical studies and data behind these claims are not that conclusive. Beyond the catastrophic warnings so frequently offered, the studies themselves contain significant small side comments and quiet caveats such as the following:

- "Maternal obesity is associated with an increased risk of stillbirth, *although the mechanisms to explain this association are not clear*" (our emphasis, Chu et al. 223).
- "The reason obese pregnant women are more likely to end up with a cesarean delivery *is not known*" (our emphasis, Leddy et al. 175).

- Studies suggest they have "confirmed the previously established association" or "found an association" or documented "yet another adverse pregnancy outcome associated with maternal obesity" (Watkins et al. 1152), but then may note "some of this association is *likely explained by other factors*" (our emphasis, Chu et al. 223).
- One study on the long-term health impact for children of obese parents, for example, notes that genetics may be one of those "other factors." Shared genes, this study argues, may account for as much as 90 percent of the difference in BMI of offspring and "needs to be considered" (O'Reilly and Reynolds 14).

A lack of "mechanisms" and "reasons" for these associations means a lack of causation, and that is a significant piece of information. Alternative factors that "need to be considered" may turn out to have causal relationships, or those relationships may be found in something else entirely, which researchers have yet to consider. Deb Burgard, a psychologist and size diversity advocate, critiques studies linking health problems with BMI; she states that these are only correlations, not causal relationship. Furthermore, she notes that those correlations are minor in the whole picture of health, and often account for a small fraction of health problems; the vast majority of health outcomes relate to factors other than BMI (43). In other words, even if those correlations turned out to have a causal relationship, BMI and size would still not be among the most significant factors affecting health. Currently, these correlations are framed as having a significant causal relationship, which serves to naturalize fatphobic beliefs and affirm the disease of obesity. If we reject fatness as a disease and affirm that people of all sizes can have healthy pregnancies and deserve compassionate prenatal care, we can direct our research and clinical efforts to developing strategies and tools for improving outcomes.

Studies on stillbirth are a prime example of an area of research where an emphasis on BMI as a risk factor is not providing useful directions for care providers or pregnant people. As noted above, studies have shown increased rates of stillbirth among overweight and obese people (Chu et al. 223), but the mechanisms to explain this association are unknown. Stillbirth affects about one in two hundred pregnancies (Spong ix), and in the majority of those cases, the cause is unrelated to BMI and remains unexplained (Fretts 8). The association of fatness with increased risk of stillbirth may be "directly related to obesity, or it could be due to associated comorbidities such as GDM ([gestational] diabetes) or hypertensive disorders" (IOG et al. 11)—both of which are also associated with higher BMIs (Leddy et al. 175). This possibility provides no greater clarity; the association of gestational diabetes with body size "has yet to be fully delineated" (177), and gestational diabetes is linked to several other demographic factors beyond fatness. Being over thirty-five years old, being Hispanic or Asian, having less than twelve years of schooling, and having your third (or more) baby are all also correlated with an increased risk for gestational diabetes (Leddy et al. 177). The association of educational level with risk reminds us that social and cultural factors are often at play in health as well as in studies of health.

Another area in which a cited risk of women with higher BMIs raises more questions than it answers is the two-to-threefold increase in Caesarean births among people over two hundred pounds. As Anna Tsing argues in the quote cited above, technology can be a vehicle for the cultural production of natural difference. This increased risk for surgical birth is a good example of this. One specific technology of birth is the external fetal monitor (EFM). Routinely used in labour, an EFM is a combination of two sensors: one using ultrasound to monitor the fetal heart rate and the other measuring the length and frequency of contractions. Research shows that continuous fetal monitoring does not improve outcomes for pregnant people or their babies (Devane et al.) and has negative impacts on labour, such as decreased mobility, increased rates of Caesarean birth, and assisted vaginal deliveries (Alfirevic et al.; ACNM). Consumer Reports lists continuous monitoring as something to "reject when you're expecting," yet it remains nearly universal on hospital labour and delivery units (Haelle).

The reasons for the increase in Caesarean birth rates among women are unknown, but some researchers cite "dysfunctional labor" as one theory (Leddy et al. 175). Dysfunctional labour generally describes "abnormal" contraction patterns and "slow" cervical dilation, as well as a labour progress that deviates from normal—all of which could be critiqued as a dysfunctional expectation for women in labour. Studies showing slower cervical dilation in women with higher BMIs also support this theory of dysfunctional labour. Although these studies do not document any reasons why dilation is slower, there is ample evidence to suggest that being restricted to a hospital bed impedes labour progress (Lawrence et al.). The American College of Gynecologists and Obstetricians (ACOG) has stated that it is more difficult to monitor the babies of fat pregnant people. This difficulty with the technology results in hospitals staff placing greater restrictions on movement during labour, which is acknowledged by ACOG as a risk for Caesarean delivery. Thus, researchers looking at the impact of obesity could be looking in the wrong place. Pregnant people are warned that their dangerous bodies and dysfunctional labour warrant more Caesarean births, but failed technology, along with poor clinical expectations, may more likely be the culprit.

Giving fat people unnecessary Caesareans puts them in danger. Caesarean births increase the risk of infection and can cause damage to organs around the uterus, heavy blood loss, and blood clots in the legs and lungs. Caesarean births also increase risks to the baby from injury during delivery as well as problems associated with being born premature (when born before thirty-nine weeks or when the due date is miscalculated). There are also slightly higher long-term risks associated with Caesarean births—including the risk of uterine rupture on the incision scar, higher rates of future placental problems, and risk of future hysterectomy. For fat people, there are also more complications during recovery from a Caesarean birth (Machado); there is also less chance of having a future vaginal birth, which compounds the risk (Leddy et al. 175). Again, these are not necessarily risks of body size per se; they may equally be risks of being a fat person in a fatphobic healthcare system.

After having an initial Caesarean birth, fat people are cautioned that their weight decreases their chances of ever having a vaginal birth with subsequent pregnancies. Researchers have concluded that people under two hundred pounds have higher rates of vaginal births after a Caesarean birth (VBAC), at about 82 percent; however, between two hundred and three hundred pounds, the success rate drops to 57 percent, and over three hundred pounds, the VBAC rate was only 13 percent (Leddy et al. 175). Yet in light of concerns with fetal monitoring and provider bias, these differences in success rates may be attributed to factors that have nothing to do with the pregnant person or their labour. Furthermore, there is huge variability in VBAC success rates among different care providers (Catling-Paull et al.). Most people are discouraged from attempting a vaginal birth (ACOG 2010), especially fat people who are already seen as risky patients with a low chance of success.

Cultural understandings of how size affects health, combined with a generalized fear of fatness, have circumscribed the questions researchers are asking and the clinical care that fat people are getting. Data on weight gain and fatness in pregnancy are riddled with assumptions not grounded in evidence. Pregnant people are being advised about risks that could be caused as much by the bias against fat people as by the fatness itself. As McCullough has noted, "perhaps the medical establishment should also be concerned about the correlation between stigmatizing treatment ... and birth outcomes" (230). McCullough poignantly states that this data may point to the dysfunction of the medical system rather than that of the fat body.

Our intention is not to suggest that there is no causal connection between eating well and staying active on the one hand, and between better outcomes in pregnancy and birth on the other hand. On the contrary, cultural preoccupations with BMI and weight gain as the cause of complications, interventions, and risks have discouraged research into what other causal relationships, and the mechanism of those risks, may more usefully improve outcomes for pregnant people and their babies. Following Metzl, we argue against the current ideologies of health, which are saturated with stigma and mask the power and privilege behind naturalized difference; we argue for science, medical research, and the ability to improve pregnancies outcomes and health. Currently, we know very little relative to what we believe we know, and this is concerning.

Sites of Resistance

In the U.S. today, at least two-thirds of pregnant people have weight gain inconsistent with the Institute of Medicine's (IOM) guidelines (Leddy et al.). This means that deviations from these guidelines, even with care providers attempting to manage weight gain during pregnancy, are actually the norm. Over one-third of Americans are clinically labelled obese, and this number appears to be growing (CDC). This fact is framed as a crisis in studies and reports, and as "a growing worldwide epidemic among women of reproductive age" (Buschur and Kim 6). Care providers are admonished that it is their moral and clinical obligation to intervene (Phelan; Stengel et al.). Yet beyond the moral panic lies the clear fact that pregnant people are not, on the whole, complying with the stated guidelines about weight gain in pregnancy. This is the material reality, and no amount of insisting that it should be different has changed this fact.

Quality care and support are essential to a healthy and positive experience of pregnancy and birth. Perceptions of care during this time—from care providers, medical staff, supports people, and partners—have long-term psychological and physical impacts. A positive birth experience increases confidence, self-efficacy, and bonding with your baby (Simpkin). Many parents have also shared that their birth had a positive impact on their body image. Pregnancy presents unique opportunities to experience the body in an entirely new way. For a person who has been shamed for their body size, growing and birthing a healthy child can be an important affirmation that their body is not broken, but strong and capable. Additionally, for individuals with a history of disordered eating and body hatred, experiencing the body as functional and food as sustenance for themselves and their growing baby can present a shift within their patterns of relating to food and body. Critical to supporting this shift is how care providers respond to these changes—whether they are affirming or shaming. The effects of this are felt well beyond the immediate postpartum time and can set the stage for a radically new way of being in one's body. Given that the majority of pregnant people are gaining weight in pregnancy at a rate beyond the guidelines and that the guidelines themselves are arbitrary and not evidence based, it is time to reevaluate the usefulness of these protocols.

Birth can be a powerful opportunity to rewrite body narratives. Despite pathologizing discourse around weight and weight gain, pregnant people of all sizes are finding ways to reclaim their dangerous pregnant bodies. These counter narratives—celebrations of body diversity in pregnancy—abound in social media and online communities. New reclamation projects offer an alternative paradigm to being pregnant and a space for new parents to share their stories that are not given a platform in mainstream depictions of pregnancy. In the Body Positive Pregnancy and Parenting Facebook group that we moderate, for example, one person wrote:

> My relationship with my body has always been centrally about both being fat and being super capable so pregnancy made me feel more fat and less capable.... [But] giving birth was such an incredible experience for me. I really did feel like I climbed Everest.... It still feels like the single greatest feat of bodily strength and I think it is a reference point of sorts, like if I could do that, I can do anything.

Other parents in the group similarly noted that giving birth made them feel strong and capable, in awe of their bodies, and more able to trust themselves.

Another example of an online community for fat pregnant people is Plus Size Birth (PSB). PSB offers educational information, size-friendly referrals, and a safe space to make connections and share stories. PSB's founder, Jen McLellan, was inspired to create this community by her own experience of birthing. She writes "On August 24, 2010 my life was forever changed by the birth of my son. On that day I not only became a mother but also developed a whole new love for my body." Her birth experience gave way to a new narrative of her body as strong and powerful, and from that, she launched a haven for those resisting pathologizing narratives about their fat, dangerous bodies.

These informal online communities among fat pregnant people mirror larger cultural trends. Fat studies scholars in academe and beyond are crafting theoretical and political interventions into current ideologies of health, understandings of body size and diversity, and approaches to medicine, dieting, and the science of size. Fat activists are organizing for the rights of fat people and seeking to end size discrimination. The Health at Every Size (HAES) movement has emerged from this political space, and could usefully be applied to prenatal care rather than the current weight-centred model that shames people for their risky bodies.

Despite the overwhelming clinical and cultural belief that fat bodies are dangerous and weight gain in pregnancy is the problem, people of all sizes give birth to healthy babies every day. HAES offers a model that moves away from ideal weights and target BMI ranges, and embraces a weight-neutral paradigm that honours size diversity and focuses on behaviours over numbers. Deb Burgard, psychologist and HAES co-founder, describes this approach as "a commitment to assessing clients and patients on an individual basis, and rejecting the conventional assumption that arbitrary BMI dividing lines ('overweight,' 'obese') are indications of pathology in individuals" (49). Although providers across the country are beginning to adopt this framework into their practice, it is largely absent from prenatal healthcare and is badly needed.

Currently, care providers are instructed to address weight and diet without having the tools to navigate these conversations; they are left to rely on their own personal understandings of nutrition and weight. Because of this, it is not uncommon for pregnant people to receive confusing and non-evidence-based nutritional advice. Instead of relying on BMI and scales, care providers would do better to begin with certain questions. For example—how are you feeling?; how are you feeding yourself?; are you eating to hunger and stopping when full?; are you eating nutrient-dense foods?; are you getting enough protein in your diet and eating ample amounts of vegetables?; are you getting regular physical activity?; and do you feel good physically, emotionally? These questions would give care providers opportunities to have meaningful conversations with their patients about health and wellness and the importance of caring for themselves during pregnancy. More so, they would provide an important space for pregnant people to practice a new way of thinking about and caring for their body—one not dictated by external guidelines or a number on the scale. The impacts of this shift extend well beyond the months of pregnancy and postpartum; they have the potential to set the foundation for raising children who too will have healthy relationships to food and body.

Conclusion

Fat people give birth to healthy babies every single day in this country, and many more could with appropriate care (Viraday, "Reply"). Similarly, thin people have complicated pregnancies every day, and they too could have healthier pregnancies with appropriate care. There may be health consequences connected to fatness in pregnancy (though the connections remain unclear), but shaming people and relying on BMI, scales, and unfounded dieting advice as primary tools for predicting risk are not improving health or outcomes. Even if fatness were a proven risk (which it is not), fat people deserve appropriate prenatal care informed by the best evidence and practised in dialogue with patients about their own behaviours and health. A cultural bias against fat people has created a healthcare system in which the ability to care for all people is hindered by an unfounded belief that size is a good indicator of overall health and risk. This belief affects every facet of care offered to pregnant people as well as the research around how to make all pregnancies healthier.

Preoccupations with weight and body size in prenatal care continue to fuel dangerous and exclusive narratives of parenthood and motherhood. Prenatal care identifies healthy and good reproducing bodies while it pathologizes those bodies that do not abide by the norm (i.e., thinness) as risky to the baby. Putnam's New York Times article details every crisis and complication she's seen with obese and "super obese" clients in her work as an obstetrician. She details the challenge fat patients pose to doctors who could be injured treating large patients and calls for "creating special labour and delivery centres for severely obese patients that are equipped with automatic lifts, specially designed monitors and appropriately trained teams." This is not the direction prenatal care in this country should take. Appropriately trained care providers and technology that can accommodate all people are certainly needed, but further alienating and stigmatizing fat people in special high-risk centres is not the way to accomplish that.

We do have a healthcare crisis in this country: we spend more money on prenatal and postpartum healthcare than any other country in the world, yet we rank sixtieth in pregnancy-related mortality globally (CIC). But the solution to this crisis will not be found in more interventions and greater stigmatization of fat pregnant people. We need to shift away from a model that treats pregnant bodies as obstacles to the health and safety of unborn children (as well as to themselves, their doctors, and the nation). We must move toward a model encouraging health in all pregnancies at all sizes. Fatphobia, naturalized as a health crisis, has only decreased the health of fat parents while increasing the number of unnecessary and unsafe interventions. We need to reimagine prenatal care models that will improve the health and safety of all people, regardless of size.

Endnotes

1 Borrowing from fat activists, such as Marilyn Wann, we use the term fat rather than the clinical terms "obese" and "overweight" to reclaim the word as a neutral adjective and political identity (xii).

2 Tsipy Ivry's analysis of prenatal care in Japan and Israel exemplifies how weight gain in pregnancy is monitored and managed in other cultures. She notes that in both cases, weight was routinely monitored by care providers, but "Japanese practitioners are even more concerned that their American counterparts with the dimensions of the pregnant body" while "Israeli ob-gyns ... paid relatively little attention to weight-gain monitoring" (70). She reads this difference as an "expression of medical authority" born out of different "cultural paradigms for thinking about pregnancy, women, and fetuses, and not necessarily with hard numbers (whose meanings and the methods through which they are manufactures should be always carefully considered)" (74).

3 It is also worth noting that within these studies there are enormous variations in how size and risk are being defined and delineated. Many of the best studies on maternal obesity are meta-analysis drawn from a wide variety of clinical contexts and research projects, bundled together to assess risks and outcomes. Although this is useful in that is offers a larger data set to potentially strengthen the integrity of the results, it also means that different indexes have been used to define what constitutes overweight or obese. (BMI and weight in pounds are both variously used and within each, different numbers are the cut off for being considered obese or overweight.) Thus the data can also be questionable because of this cross-study variability and lack of consistency in classification.

Works Cited

American College of Obstetricians and Gynecologists (ACOG). "Ob Gyns Issue Less Restrictive VBAC Guidelines." *Practice Bulletin: Clinical Management Guidelines for Obstetricians-Gynecologists,* vol. 116, no. 2, 2010, pp. 450-63.

American College of Nurse-Midwives (ACNM). "Intermittent Auscultation for Intrapartum Fetal Heart Rate Surveillance: Clinical

Bulletin No. 11." *Journal of Midwifery & Women's Health*, vol. 55, no 4, 2010, pp. 397-403.

Alfirevic, Zarko, et al. "Continuous Cardiotocography (CTG) as a Form of Electronic Fetal Monitoring (EFM) for Fetal Assessment during Labour." *Cochrane Database of Systematic Reviews*, 2017, www.cochrane.org/CD006066/PREG_continuous-cardiotocography-ctg-form-electronic-fetal-monitoring-efm-fetal-assessment-during-labour. Accessed 18 July 2018.

Bacon, Linda. *Health at Every Size: The Surprising Truth about your Weight*. BenBella Books Inc., 2008.

Burgard, Deb. "What is Health at Every Size?" *The Fat Studies Reader*, edited by Esther Rothblum and Sondra Solovay, NYU Press, 2009, pp. 42-53.

Buscher, Elizabeth, and Catherine Kim. "Guidelines and Interventions for Obesity During Pregnancy." *International Journal of Gynecology and Obstetrics*, vol. 119, no. 1, 2012, pp. 6-10.

Campos, Paul, et al. "The Epidemiology of Overweight and Obesity: Public Health Crisis or Moral Panic?" *International Journal of Epidemiology*, vol. 35, no. 1, 2006, pp. 55-60.

Chu, Susan Y, et al. "Maternal Obesity and risk of stillbirth: A Meta Analysis." *American Journal of Obstetrics and Gynecology*, vol. 197, no. 3, 2008, pp. 223-28.

Haelle, Tara. "Childbirth: What to Reject When You're Expecting. 9 Procedures to Think Twice about during Your Pregnancy." *Consumer Reports*, 2017, www.consumerreports.org/pregnancy-childbirth/childbirth-what-to-reject-when-youre-expecting/. Accessed 18 July 2018.

Devane, Declan, et al. "Cardiotocography versus intermittent Auscultation of fetal heart on admission of labour ward for assessment of fetal wellbeing." *Cochrane Database of Systematic Reviews*, vol. 1, 2017, pp. 1-46, doi: 10.1002/14651858.CD005122.pub5.

Fretts, Ruth. "High Income Countries." *Stillbirth: Prediction, Prevention, and Management*, edited by Catherine Spong, Wiley-Black-well Publishing, 2011, pp. 3-18.

Guggenheim, Jez A, et al. "Myopia, Genetics, and Ambient Lighting at Night in a UK Sample." *British Journal of Ophthalmology*, vol. 85, no. 5, 2003, pp. 580-82.

Institute of Obstetricians and Gynecologists (IOG). "Obesity and Pregnancy Clinical Practice Guideline." *Institute of Obstetricians and*

Gynecologists, vol. 1, no. 2, 2013, pp. 1-39.

Ivry, Tsipy. *Embodying Culture: Pregnancy in Japan and Israel.* Rutgers University Press, 2009.

Klein, Richard. "What Is Health and How Do You Get It?" *Against Health: How Health Became the New Morality,* edited by Jonathan Michael Metzl and Anna Kirkland, New York University Press, 2010, pp. 15-25.

Lawlor, Debbie, et al. "Commentary: The Hormone Replacement-Coronary Heart Disease Conundrum: Is This the Death of Observational Epidemiology?" *International Journal of Epidemiology,* vol. 33, no. 3, 2004, pp. 464-67.

Lawrence, Annamarie, et al. "Maternal positions and mobility during first stage labour."

Cochrane Database of Systematic Reviews, vol. 10, 2013, pp. 1-96, doi: 10.1002/14651858.CD003934.pub4 LeBesco, Kathleen. "Fat Panic and the New Morality." *Against Health: How Health Became the New Morality,* edited by Jonathan Michael Metzl and Anna Kirkland, New York University, Press, 2010, pp. 72-83.

Leddy, Meaghan A, et al. "The Impact of Maternal Obesity on Maternal and Fetal Health." *Reviews in Obstetrics & Gynecology,* vol. 1, no. 4, 2008, pp. 170-78.

Machado, Lovina. "Cesarean Section in Morbidly Obese Parturients: Practical Implications and Complications." *North American Journal of Medical Sciences,* vol. 4, no. 1, 2012, pp. 13-18.

Martin, Emily. "The Egg and The Sperm: How Science Has Constructed a Romance Based on Stereotypical Male-Female." *Signs,* vol. 16, no. 3, 1990, pp. 485-501.

Martin, Emily. *The Woman in the Body: A Cultural Analysis of Reproduction.* Beacon Press, 1992.

Mayo Clinic. "Pregnancy and Obesity: Know the Risks." *Mayo Clinic,* 2018, www.mayoclinic.org/healthy-lifestyle/pregnancy-week-by-week/in-depth/pregnancy-and-obesity/art-20044409. Accessed 18 Juy 2018.

Metzl, Jonathan, and Anna Kirkland, editors. *Against Health: How Health Became the New Morality.* New York University Press, 2010.

McCullough, Megan. "Fat and Knocked Up: An Embodied Analysis of Stigma, Visibility, and Invisibility in the Biomedical Management of an Obese Pregnancy." *Reconstructing Obesity: The Meaning of Measures and the Measure of Meanings,* edited by Megan B.

McCullough and Jessica A. Hardin, Berghahn Books, 2013, pp. 215-34.

McLellan, Jen. "Meet Jen McLellan." *Plus Size Birth*, 2018, plussizebirth.com/jen-mclellan/. Accessed 18 July 2018.

Institute of Medicine (IOM) and National Research Council (NRC). *Weight Gain During Pregnancy: Reexamining the Guidelines*. The National Academies Press, 2009.

Nuthalapaty, Francis S, et al. "The Association of Maternal Weight with Cesarean Risk, Labor Duration, and Cervical Dilation Rate during Labor Induction." *Obstetrics and Gynecology*, vol. 103, no. 3, 2004, pp. 452-56.

O'Reilly, JR, and RM Reynolds. "The Risk of Maternal Obesity to the Long-Term Health of the Offspring." *Clinical Endocrinology-Oxford*, vol. 78, no. 1, 2013, pp. 9-16.

Oster, Emily. *Expecting Better: Why Conventional Pregnancy Wisdom is Wrong and What You Really Need to Know*. Penguin Books, 2014.

Phelan, Suzanne. "Pregnancy: A 'Teachable Moment' for Weight Control and Obesity Prevention." *American Journal of Obstetrics and Gynecology*, vol. 202, no. 2, 2010, pp. 1-16.

Putnam, Claire. "Pregnant, Obese...and in Danger." *New York Times*, 2015, www.nytimes.com/2015/03/29/opinion/sunday/pregnant-obese-and-in-danger.html. Accessed 18 July 2018.

Quinn, Graham, et al. "Myopia and Ambient Lighting at Night." *Nature*, vol. 399, 1999, pp. 113-14.

Saw SM, et al. "Near-Work Activity, Night-Lights, and Myopia in the Singapore-China Study." *Archives of Ophthalmology*, vol. 120, no. 5, 2002, pp. 620-27.

Spong, Catherine, editor. *Stillbirth: Prediction, Prevention, and Management*. Wiley-Blackwell Publishing, 2011.

Stengel, Michael, et al. "'What My Doctor Didn't Tell Me': Examining Health Care Provider

Advice to Overweight and Obese Pregnant Women on Gestational Weight Gain and Physical Activity." *Women's Health Issues*, vol. 22, no. 6, 2012, pp. 535-40.

Tsing, Anna Lowenhaupts. "Empowering Nature, or: Some Gleanings in Bee Culture." *Naturalizing Power: Essays in Feminist Cultural Analysis*, edited by Sylvia Junko Yanagisako and Carol Delaney, Routledge, 1995, pp. 113-43.

Vahratian, Anjel, et al. "Maternal Prepregnancy Overweight and Obesity and the Pattern of Labor Progression in Term Nulliparous Women." *Obstetrics and Gynecology*, vol. 104, no. 5, 2004, pp. 943-51.

Viraday, Pamela. "Reply Turned Post: Ghettoizing Fat Pregnant Women." *Well Rounded Mama*, 2009, wellroundedmama.blogspot.com/2009/12/reply-turned-post-ghettoizing-fat.html. Accessed 25 July 2018.

Viraday, Pamela. "The Fat Vagina Theory: 'Soft Tissue Dystocia.'" *Well Rounded Mama*, 2010, https://wellroundedmama.blogspot.com/2010/12/fat-vagina-theory-soft-tissue-dystocia.html. Accessed 25 July 2018.

Watkins, ML, et al. "Maternal Obesity and the Risk for Birth Defects." *Pediatrics*, vol. 111, no. 1, 2003, pp. 1152-158.

Wann, Marilyn. "Foreward." *The Fat Studies Reader*, edited by Esther Rothblum and Sondra Solovay. New York University Press, 2009, pp. xi-xxvii.

Yanagisako, Sylvia, and Carol Delaney, editors. *Naturalizing Power: Essays in Feminist Cultural Analysis*. Routledge, 1995.

Zadnik K, et al. "Myopia and ambient night-time lighting." *Nature*, vol. 404, no. 6774, 2000, pp. 143-44.

Zolotor, AJ, and MC Carlough. "Update on Prenatal Care." *American Family Physician*, vol. 89, no. 3, 2014, pp. 199-208.

Chapter Three

"Consideration of the Unborn Child": Advance Directives and Pregnancy Exclusion Laws

Claire Marguerite Leonard Horn

The "right to die" was introduced as a legal principle in New Jersey in 1976. In a courtroom heavily populated by media and concerned citizens, Karen Ann Quinlan's parents argued against two doctors, a court-appointed guardian, and a hospital lawyer for permission to unplug the machines that were keeping their vegetative daughter alive. In 1990, nearly fourteen years after the Quinlan court ruled in her parents' favour, Allison August and Steven Miles conducted a study of right-to-die cases in the United States. They examined the twenty-two right-to-die decisions that had occurred in America. Following suspicions aroused by the paternalistic fervour surrounding the Quinlan case, they coded for distinctions between the fourteen cases involving women and the eight cases involving men. Their work indicated significant disparities between the court's willingness to accept evidence on the end-of-life preferences of female patients in these cases, and their willingness to accept evidence about male patient preferences. In "six of the eight cases involving men without advance directives, appellate courts constructed the patient's own preference for medical treatment from the memories and insights of family and friends" (August and Miles 86). By contrast, the court only constructed preference for women in two of fourteen cases. Where preferences were constructed for these two women only because of "very specific remarks they made about medical treatment" (89), the cases in which constructed preferences for men were allowed "incorporated evidence ranging from specific discussions, to general discussions remote from the time and possibility of illness to constructions simply based on the man's character" (89). Beyond this apparent bias in the court's acceptance of constructed preferences, August and Miles note that the language used by judges in these cases reflected an understanding of women's previous remarks to family and friends as childish or uninformed, whereas men's comments were treated as reflective of "mature, rational choice[s]" (87). Since August and Miles completed their study, other academics across disciplines—including Robin Fiore, Karla Holloway, and Katherine Taylor—have considered and critiqued emergent patterns with regard to how gendered biases operate in judicial and medical discourse on the right to die.

Following Katherine Taylor, I am interested in the unique circumstances of cases involving pregnant women. Although the likelihood of any individual falling into a persistent vegetative state or becoming braindead remains low, examining the legal and medical discourse that emerges around right-to-die cases that centre on pregnant patients in the United States remains a useful practice in several regards. First, the laws and policies that currently exist around such cases place direct limitations on the rights of all women as patients. Second, analyzing common practice in these cases reveals problematic social expectations about motherhood and maternal responsibility as well as the ways that medical and legal institutions amplify and enforce these expectations.

Every American patient is encouraged to file advance directives when registering with a new doctor or preparing for any significant medical procedure. Advance directives include living will documents, which allow patients to specify their wishes for medical treatment in the event of an emergency, and power of attorney documents, which allow patients to name a family member or friend to enact these wishes for them and make treatment decisions on their behalf. When a medical emergency occurs and the patient has left advance directives, hospitals are legally required to follow these directives, except if a patient is pregnant. Pregnancy exclusion laws are statutes that exist in nearly every American state, and stipulate that the applicability of women's advance directives will be limited in the event of pregnancy. In most states, these statutes explicitly prohibit a woman's advance directives from being honoured should she become incapacitated even a few days into a pregnancy. Given that advance directives written by any person when medically competent are legally binding except where a patient is pregnant, these statutes convey that the law views pregnant women—and women who may file a living will or power of attorney document with the knowledge they could become pregnant—as incompetent.

Where these laws inhibit the termination of a pregnancy before fetal viability (between twenty-four and twenty-six weeks), as they do in many states, they are in express conflict with *Roe v. Wade*, which protects American women's access to abortion prior to fetal viability (Greene and Wolfe 1). *Roe v. Wade* grants that the state's interest in the survival of the fetus does not outweigh interest in protecting a woman's privacy until after the fetus is viable. Pregnancy exclusions that specify that a pregnant woman with a previable fetus cannot be removed from life support (even when she has explicitly specified in an advance directive that she does not want life-sustaining measures taken) directly violate the stipulation in Roe that prior to viability, a woman's right to private choice is to be protected. They also negate her ability to articulate the manner and extent to which she wishes medical intervention on her own body to occur, and to specify how her wishes may change in the event of pregnancy. Would she want any possible measures taken to save a nearly viable fetus but none taken if—as in many cases—the fetus had almost no chance of survival? Who would she want to speak for her and her baby if she was unable to? Would she choose to leave this decision to her partner, or to someone more removed? Would she find the concept of becoming an incubator following her death so repugnant as to refuse any extraordinary measures?

Pregnancy exclusion laws do not allow any woman—regardless of how pressing such a possibility may be in her circumstances—to make these decisions. Instead, they presume that the most appropriate decision makers are doctors or lawyers acting on behalf of the state. Although several end-of-life cases involving pregnant women have occurred in the past few years, I use the Marlise Munoz case, heard in 2014, in order to analyze how these issues manifest in real life. Although many interesting bioethical questions could be raised here, my approach is a legal analysis of the arguments made in Munoz. I have adopted this methodology to begin to unpack how American sociocultural understandings of motherhood and pregnancy are mobilized in this case, and to consider how courts frame women such as Munoz in order to justify state intervention. Building on Munoz and considering the broader reach of these laws, I suggest that pregnancy exclusions should be understood as a way for the state to exert control over a woman's body by extending power over her life beyond her death.

Munoz as a Wayward Mother

On 26 November 2013, paramedic Marlise Munoz, who was fourteen weeks pregnant, collapsed in her home in Texas. Two days later, she was declared braindead by John Peter Smith Hospital. Her husband, Erick Munoz, with the support of her parents, requested that life support be withdrawn. The hospital refused on the grounds of Munoz's pregnancy, and the case went to court. As Erick Munoz's lawyers argued, "Erick and Marlise worked as paramedics during their marriage, and thus were knowledgeable of and had personally witnessed injuries that resulted in death, including brain death" (qtd. in *Munoz v. John Peter Smith Hospital* 3). Given their regular exposure to these realities, Erick Munoz's legal team argued that both knew to "express clearly to each other, family members, and friends, their respective desires not to be resuscitated should either of them become brain dead" (3). Erick Munoz established that Marlise Munoz had told him, their friends, and her parents on countless occasions that she "did not want to be kept on life sustaining measures" (2). Due to Marlise Munoz's pregnancy, however, neither John Peter Smith Hospital nor the court was concerned with acknowledging what Marlise Munoz's end-of-life wishes may have been. Under Section 166.001 of the Texas Health and Safety Act, "a person may not withdraw or withhold life-sustaining treatment...from a pregnant patient," meaning that in situations like the one Marlise Munoz was in, physicians are legally required to ignore any previously expressed wishes of the mother and to do everything in their power to sustain her or else face legal consequences.

Although at the time of the trial in which Erick Munoz challenged John Peter Smith Hospital to remove his wife's respirator the hospital and lawyers on both sides of the case agreed that the "fetus gestating inside Mrs. Munoz [was] not viable" (qtd. in *Munoz* 2) at the time of the trial, the case proceeded with the legal team for the hospital insisting that regardless of the wishes of Marlise Munoz or her family, the state had a "commitment to protect unborn children" (qtd.in *Munoz* 4) and thus should not allow Munoz to die. As both Munoz's team and the defense team for John Peter Smith Hospital recognized, at the time of the Munoz trial "There [was] no case law interpreting" (2) how the pregnancy exclusion in the Health and Safety Act might be applied to a situation involving a braindead pregnant woman.

In previous right-to-die cases involving women, researchers have observed a pattern wherein courts frame these patients as vulnerable and in need of protection. In their study, August and Miles found that "courts explicitly claimed a parental role only in relation to females (Cruzan; Quinlan); such a role was specifically rejected in the case of a male" (196). Where courts attribute self-determination to male patients regardless of whether a judge can imagine these patients as their son, father, or brother, women are read and framed in these cases as relational objects. These scenarios expose "social expectations that, for the sake of others, women should forego acting on interests they may have in relieving their suffering by hastening death" (Fiore 195). In assessing what is right for female patients according to their relationships with others rather than their previously expressed wishes, courts interpellate women as something belonging to the people around them rather than as subjects who might have had their own "interests" in the kind of treatment they receive.

In some cases, such as Schiavo and Quinlan,[1] the patients have been positioned in relation to their parents; however, Munoz, as a pregnant woman, is understood as a mother first, not as an individual. Whereas Quinlan and Schiavo were framed as being in need of state protection, Munoz is framed as a wayward mother, from whom the state must protect a child. Penelope Deutscher refers to the way in which "the woman legally forbidden to have an abortion is sometimes figured as a potentially murderous competing sovereign whose self-interest would thwart the intervening motivations of the state" (66). In Deutscher's estimation, women who seek abortions are discussed in political and legal discourse as though they are trying to gain the power to kill a child, and they will succeed unless the state intervenes. Munoz was not a conscious woman actively seeking an abortion, yet in the medical and judicial discourse surrounding her case, this same kind of frame—Munoz as a potentially murderous woman whom the state must prevent from terminating a child—is evident.

The framing of Munoz as a bad mother trying to take the life of the fetus from beyond the grave is present in the language used by the legal team who represented John Peter Smith Hospital. Responding to Erick Munoz's first argument on behalf of his wife—that the law forbidding the removal of life-sustaining measures from a pregnant patient did not apply because "Marlise Munoz [was] legally dead under Texas law" (*Munoz* 4) and "a life sustaining measure cannot apply to the dead"—the JPS legal team state that his response "ignores consideration of the unborn child" (2). Here, the defense team deliberately choose language to present the fetus as an already existing human being, not as a fetus, not even as an unborn infant, but as an unborn child. In choosing this language, the JPS team echoes a broader antiabortion discourse. Although under current jurisprudence a previable fetus is not a person, choosing to call it a "child" rather than a "fetus" invokes the spectre of an already existing child being killed rather than a fetus being terminated.

The JPS team conceded Erick Munoz's argument that Marlise Munoz was legally dead, yet it held that to suggest it was wrong to sustain her on a machine was to make a decision that was unjust to the fetus. Although Munoz's fetus was well before viability (which is legally placed at around twenty-four weeks) and medical evidence suggests that a fetus at such a stage could not grow without nutrients from a live mother, the JPS team referenced the Texas Woman's Right to Know Act. They cited the following principles of this act—that "substantial medical evidence recognizes that an unborn child is capable of experiencing pain by not later than twenty weeks after fertilization" (4), and that "the state has a compelling interest in protecting the lives of unborn children from the stage at which substantial medical evidence indicates that these children are capable of feeling pain" (4). Although the Woman's Right to Know Act could not apply to a fetus at fourteen weeks, referencing this language introduced the idea that to remove Munoz from life support was to cause actual injury to a child. After creating this framework, it was possible for the JPS lawyers to make the claim that "the State has clearly expressed its desire to protect the life of unborn children" and that therefore it was "unreasonable to argue that the State intended to forgo its interest in the life and welfare of the unborn child upon the death of the mother" (4).

This discursive figuring disassociates the fetus from Marlise Munoz, as though she has ceded motherly duties by dying and the court has a responsibility to intervene and ensure that the baby is cared for. This framing of Munoz as a kind of "bad mother" is reinforced by the defendants' claim that the Texas statute preventing life support from being removed from a pregnant patient "must convey legislative intent to protect the unborn child, otherwise the legislature would have simply allowed a pregnant patient to decide to let her life, and the life of her unborn child, end" (qtd. in *Munoz* 3).

Here, the argument is made that the pregnancy exclusion must be honoured even if the mother is dead. The language of choice is invoked to suggest that if it is not honoured in these cases, the state might as well permit "a pregnant patient to decide to let her life ... ...end." The implication in using the word "decide" is that to not extend the pregnancy exclusion to cases where the mother is dead is akin to the state allowing the suicide of pregnant mothers, allowing them to "decide" to end their lives and those of their fetuses. Despite the fact that Munoz was unconscious and legally dead, Erick Munoz's argument for removing the respirator that was sustaining her is framed here as an argument in favour of a mother "allowing" her child to die. Although Marlise Munoz was in no way responsible for her brain-dead state, JPS used language that raised the spectre of the suicide of a pregnant woman, and in doing so, suggested that Munoz made a choice to "let her life, and the life of her unborn child, end." As Deutscher writes, "in an uncanny ghosting, it is not uncommon for extreme antiabortion activists to make connections between abortion and extermination" (66).

Although the lawyers for John Peter Smith Hospital might not be defined as extreme antiabortionists, and Munoz is not an abortion case, to frame letting Munoz die as an act that would "allow" mothers to end the lives of their babies is to draw parallels between her situation and the extermination of children. The striking difference between the Munoz case and an abortion case is that the central figure wanted to be a mother, but due to circumstances entirely beyond her control, her life ended. In an abortion case, it would be patently unconstitutional for a medical professional to go to court to prevent the termination of an unwanted pregnancy prior to viability. Because the Munoz case involves a previable fetus, it is reasonable to assume that medical and legal interference in the Munoz family's choice to discontinue treatment (based on what they believed Marlise Munoz would want) would be equally unconstitutional. Yet the difficulty of end-of-life cases involving pregnant women lies in their uneasy link to *Roe v. Wade*. Where a court could not constitutionally intervene in a woman seeking a medically approved abortion of a previable fetus, a court can intervene in the termination of a previable fetus in a vegetative or braindead woman under the purview of pregnancy exclusion laws. In doing so, as I will discuss, courts could ultimately build case law in the interest of dismantling *Roe v. Wade*.

The Reach of Pregnancy Exclusions

The Texas pregnancy exclusion law, which complicated the Munoz case, is representative of statutes that exist across the United States and restrict pregnant women's end-of-life decision making. Under the Patient Self-Determination Act of 1991, hospitals, nursing homes, home health agencies, and hospices are required to inform competent adults that they have a right to prepare an advance directive. These directives include living wills (documents in which individuals can specify their preferences for end of life care) and medical proxy or power of attorney documents (which allow an individual to designate a person to make medical decisions for them in the event of an accident). As Robin Fiore writes, "In states with living will statutes, 32 of 47 limit the applicability of living wills if a woman is pregnant, explicitly prohibiting the termination of life support whether or not the fetus is viable" (198). In a study undertaken in 2012, Megan Greene and Leslie Wolfe found that "currently twelve state statutes ... automatically invalidate a woman's advance directive if she is pregnant" (3), while under the Uniform Rights of the Terminally Ill Act, fourteen states require that "life-sustaining treatment may not be withdrawn from a woman who is known to be pregnant if it is probable that the fetus will develop to the point of live birth with continuation of treatment, regardless of the woman's expressed desires to the contrary" (Greene and Wolfe 4).

In fourteen states, the law is silent regarding pregnancy at the end of life—such decisions will either be made privately, or will come to light if and when a conflict is raised (Greene and Wolfe 4). In four states, the law uses a viability standard, so that if a woman's pregnancy is pre-viability (twenty-four weeks), her declarations may apply, but if she is past viability, these preferences will automatically be overridden (4). In only five states—New Jersey, Maryland, Minnesota, Oklahoma, and Vermont—does the law allow women to specify whether and how they would want their advance directives to be altered if they were pregnant (4). As Greene and Wolfe write, these states are "models" in this field, in that they allow a woman to have "control over her body under all circumstances and protect her rights as a patient" (4).

Women between the approximate ages of twenty to forty, while possibly interested in having children, are unlikely to have filed an advance directive unless they have been given specific cause to do so—such as a life-threatening illness or a death in the family. As a result, they may not even realize that their end-of-life wishes could be ignored should they become pregnant. Greene and Wolfe note that "one of the biggest problems with pregnancy exclusions is that there is virtually no public awareness that they exist" (6). And although the growth of medical technology makes it increasingly likely that young people could find themselves in a situation where their end-of-life wishes become significant, these concepts remain remote for most people.

These statutes not only raise concerns under *Roe v. Wade* and subsequent case law by undermining the privacy rights meant to protect abortion access, they also actively "plac[e] the rights of a fetus above those of a woman" (Greene and Wolfe 7). As Taylor writes, with the continued existence of pregnancy exclusions, "women are rendered a different class of persons with lesser rights, in many states from the earliest stage of pregnancy" (51). The implications of these statues figuring women as daughters, mothers, and wives as opposed to individuals are evident in both courts and hospitals. It is the doctors and administrators who staff hospitals who most frequently raise objections to termination in right-to-die cases. As end-of-life decisions for pregnant women are placed in the hands of physicians, it is "only the rare hospital [that] would allow the withdrawal of life support from a pregnant woman" (Taylor 50) with pregnancy exclusion statutes as they now stand. If this is true in instances where physicians want to support the family's wishes but fear legal repercussions, it becomes even more problematic when a physician does not support the family's wish to remove life support.

Where the statutes in states which automatically invalidate pregnant women's advance directives are explicitly discriminatory, those where treatment cannot be withdrawn if there is probability of a live birth place physicians in a position where they "take the place of the Legislature in determining the meaning of such terms as 'probable' and 'viability'" (Greene and Wolfe 7). This leaves room for medical professionals to intervene at their discretion due to their own moral concerns, regardless of what stage of pregnancy a woman is in. The term "viability," which determines the limits of women's access to abortion under *Roe v. Wade*, is highly contentious, and has frequently sparked debate between the general public, physicians, and the law. Yet as Anne Lederman writes, "even assuming viability ought to constitute when the state's interest in the fetus's potential life outweighs the mother's autonomy and bodily integrity, the pregnancy clause denies the declarant that extent of protection" (6).

Except in the five states where pregnancy exclusions use viability as the rule, and the five where women can specify their preferences in the event of pregnancy, pregnancy exclusion statutes are in direct conflict with *Roe v. Wade*'s protections. In the Munoz case, the hospital's lawyers argued that it was unreasonable to claim that these statutes were unconstitutional or in conflict with *Roe v. Wade*. They made the argument that "The State has an unqualified interest in the preservation of human life [and] given that interest, it is reasonable to distinguish between a pregnant patient and a patient who is not pregnant" (*Munoz* 6). Although the Texas court ultimately found in favour of Erick Munoz, it did so because it was not clear whether the language in Texas's pregnancy exclusion statute applied to a braindead woman. The court refused to question the constitutionality of the statute.

As of winter 2015, lobbyists in Texas have succeeded in clarifying the language of the statute to ensure that there will be no further debate about whether it applies to braindead individuals. Under the amended statute, pregnant women's advance directives will be entirely void in circumstances of both brain death and persistent vegetative state, and a guardian ad litem and attorney will automatically be assigned to the fetus, regardless of the woman's gestational stage. In some cases, depending on the financial resources of the mother and her family, this could mean that a previable fetus has legal representation while the mother has none. In response to the Munoz finding, several other states have begun to revisit the language of their own statutes. In June 2014, Louisiana became the first to pass an amendment establishing that even a braindead woman who is newly pregnant must be sustained on life support.

What makes these laws all the more problematic is that the necessary prerequisites for a woman to challenge their constitutionality in court are near impossible. In Seattle in 1984, a woman named Joann DiNino attempted to file an advance directive with her physician. She ignored the note that stipulated her directive wouldn't apply if she were pregnant and wrote that her preferences would still hold in this situation. Even though her physician refused to accept the directive for fear of liability, he agreed to challenge the constitutionality of the Seattle pregnancy statute with her. Their case was dismissed from the court on the grounds that since DiNino was neither pregnant nor in a vegetative state, she had no standing to question the laws. The dissenting trial judges acknowledged that if the court did not hear these issues in cases like DiNino's, it was hard to imagine a situation in which they could. Even if DiNino had been pregnant, because she was healthy, she would not have been able to establish that the statutes directly harmed her, and her case would likely have been dismissed. DiNino was told to try to find a physician who would be willing to file the directive with her note on pregnancy (*DiNino v. State of Washington*). These restrictions place women in an insurmountable double bind: in order to contest these discriminatory statutes, they must be pregnant and vegetative, but if they were pregnant and vegetative, they would be unable to articulate the harm that these directives caused them.

In thirty-two states, pregnancy exclusion clauses undermine the rights of any woman who may intend to become pregnant and may want to leave directives for her end-of-life preferences. No such clause exists that so disproportionately impacts men, yet women cannot address this discrepancy in court. These laws, in their explicit nature, enact state control over women's bodies at the intersection of medicine and law more so than any other aspect of right-to-die cases.

Pregnancy Exclusions and State Control

The justification used to defend both the court's problematic framing of Munoz as a wayward mother, and the limitations placed on women's end-of-life rights by pregnancy exclusions is the survival of a baby. It is necessary to come back to a key point in the Munoz trial to begin to think about the factors at work behind this claim to be acting in the interests of preserving life. In reflecting on this justification, we must consider that even as the state fought to maintain Munoz on life support to gestate the fetus, there was no real expectation that it would survive.

Lawyers on both sides of the case indicated at the time of the hearing that the gestating fetus was not viable. Although the attorneys may have hoped that the fetus could grow to viability, given that the mother was dead, it was likely that the fetus's survival and continued growth were compromised. Other evidence that might have been expected to impact the state's interest in sustaining Munoz was the medical confirmation that the fetus had been and would continue to be negatively impacted by her condition. In a statement released by the Munoz legal team, Erick Munoz's attorneys wrote that doctors had performed a medical exam and found that "The fetus suffer[ed] from hydrocephalus [water on the brain]" and its "lower extremities [were] deformed to the extent that the gender cannot be determined" (qtd. in Ford). Because the fetus had been deprived of oxygen, it also "appear[ed to have] further abnormalities, including a possible health problem, that [could not] be specifically determined due to the immobile nature of Mrs. Munoz's deceased body" (qtd. in Ford). The gestational age of the fetus, and the doctors' examination of Munoz, then, determined that the fetus was at best severely endangered and, at worst, could not survive. The medical precedent of the previous Piazzi, Torres, and Martin cases[2] (Gregorian 401; Sisti 143)—in which each fetus (all at later stages than Munoz) died while gestating in persistently vegetative or braindead mothers suggests it is nearly impossible that an early stage fetus could survive inside a mother who is brain dead.

Although all participants in the Munoz case acknowledged that the fetus was not viable, though it showed signs of severe damage, and though the evidence from previous similar cases all indicated that the fetus was likely to die, the hospital and state persisted in attempting to sustain Munoz. This suggests that contrary to their claims, the actual life of a child had little to do with the state's efforts. Instead, it is necessary to look at the state's interest in Munoz herself.

It is useful to draw on Michel Foucault's writing on biopower to understand the reluctance of American courts and hospitals to allow women, even those with advance directives, to die naturally. Foucault writes, "death is power's limit, the moment that escapes it" (138). He argues that while under feudalism, it was once the case that the sovereign exercised power by taking life, under capitalism, the state exercises its power by controlling life: "A power whose highest function [is] perhaps no longer to kill, but to invest life through and through" (139). Right-to-die cases demonstrate in a very literal way how this power acts. In situations involving vegetative and braindead patients, the state, as represented by hospitals and the court, wields the power to maintain these patients on life-sustaining treatment and, thus, to extend its sovereignty over them. In allowing Marlise Munoz to die, the state cedes control over affirming life. Given the great disparity in right-to-die cases involving men that make it to court compared to those involving women, the emergent pattern is that where the state is willing to grant a certain amount of power over life to men without dispute, it is reluctant to do so for women.

Foucault writes that in the transition to modern forms of government, "it was the taking charge of life, more than the threat of death, that gave power its access even to the body" (143). Both hospitals and the court have exercised state power by intervening in such cases as Terri Schiavo's and Karen Ann Quinlan's to take charge of life and thus exert power over the body. In the Munoz case, through a framework that characterizes Munoz as a mother who ceded responsibility for her child, and through enforcing pregnancy exclusions, these institutions demonstrate the state's investment in the continued life of the fetus for more than one purpose. First, they indicate state power over the life of the fetus; and second, they use the sustenance of the fetus, particularly when there is no medical evidence that it will survive, as a way to continue to exert power over women's bodies beyond their actual deaths. If, as Foucault argues, death is the "limit" of power, pregnancy exclusion laws create a disturbing circumstance that allows the state to extend control over women beyond the grave.

The possibility that the state could extend an individual's life by arguing for the life of a fetus is one that is explicitly gendered. Just as it is evident in tracing the history of right to die cases that the state takes greater interest in intervening in cases involving women than men, it is also apparent that the question of preserving a brain-dead body in order to gestate a fetus targets women in particular. Although the language used by the court in the Munoz case suggests that the state has the greatest interest in preserving the life of the baby, the fact that the hospital and its attorneys continued to fight to maintain Munoz even after recognizing that the fetus had little to no chance of survival demonstrates a determined investment in not allowing Munoz to die.

Conclusion

Although physicians in American hospitals affected by pregnancy exclusion laws are likely aware of the implications of these laws, "there is no requirement for medical professionals to inform [patients] that their wishes may be ignored if they are pregnant" (Greene and Wolfe 3). In many states, there is also no note on the directive forms themselves to alert women to these statutes. Many women who have filed advance directives may be unaware that the preferences they establish in these forms, and the surrogates they appoint to fulfil their end-of-life wishes will have no power if they become pregnant.

The Munoz case and others like it have undermined the dignity of the women in question. They have placed the partners and families of these women in deeply traumatic situations. These cases, though, also have ripple effects that could hold frightening possibilities for American women more generally. Pregnancy exclusion laws can be easily dismissed as unlikely to affect many women in their lifetimes. Confronting laws such as these, however, is all the more necessary in the era of Trump's government.

It is through laws like pregnancy exclusion statutes, from which public attention is diverted, that cases against abortion protection can begin to build without notice. Indeed, these statutes could become "the predicate for states and the federal government to challenge the ruling in *Roe v. Wade* that "the unborn have never been recognized in the law as persons in the whole sense'" (Walen 163). By drawing on the Torres, Piazzi, Martin, and Munoz cases, in which *guardians ad litem* and legal teams were assigned to the respective women's unborn, pre-viable fetuses, a court could possibly build a case for recognizing a fetus as a person. This claim, if it were successful, could have devastating consequences for women's access to abortion. If a fetus can be recognized as a person at any stage of a pregnancy, it could have equal competing interests with the mother even while it is growing in her body.

It is through such legal tactics that rights can be quietly dismantled. It is therefore both in recognition of the traumatic effect of pregnancy exclusions on families, and in recognition of the ways in which these laws could be mobilized, that we must confront the ways in which pregnancy exclusions enact state control and negate the choices and integrity of pregnant women and mothers.

Endnotes

1 *In re Quinlan,* decided by the New Jersey Supreme Court in 1976, was a landmark right-to-die case in which the patient was a young woman in her twenties. Her parents fought against her doctors for the right to remove her from life support. The court initially took guardianship from her parents and placed her in the care of an outside party. The Supreme Court ultimately found that this was unconstitutional, and set the precedent for right-to-die patients and their families to be protected by the right to privacy. *Schindler v. Schiavo* is arguably the most significant right-to-die case in U.S. history. Terri Schiavo became vegetative at twenty-six, and her parents fought against her husband for nearly fifteen years as her husband sought to have her life support removed. The court ultimately decided in the husband's favour in 2005.

2 In *Piazzi,* Donna Piazzi became braindead at sixteen weeks of pregnancy. Piazzi's partner and legal guardian requested that life support be terminated, but a second man who claimed to be father requested it be maintained (Gregorian 402). The court ordered, based on "state interest in preserving potential life" (402), that Piazzi be sustained until the baby could be delivered. The baby died shortly after. In *Torres,* Susan Torres became braindead at seventeen weeks. Her husband felt she would want to be sustained on life support, and the court ordered that she be sustained until the fetus could be delivered. The fetus died at twenty-seven weeks (402). In *Martin,* Tammy Martin became vegetative after an accident at fifteen weeks of pregnancy (Sisti 143). Her family members fought her

husband to have her life support removed, as they believed that this is what she would have wanted (143). The court granted her husband guardianship, but allowed life support to be removed after the fetus died several weeks later.

Works Cited

Deutscher, Penelope. "The Inversion of Exceptionality: Foucault, Agamben, and 'Reproductive Rights.'" *South Atlantic Quarterly*, vol. 107, no. 1, 2008, pp. 55-70.

DiNino v. State of Washington. 102 Wn.2d 327. The Supreme Court of Washington, 1984. *ThaddeusPope*, www.thaddeuspope.com/images/Dinino_Wash_1984_.pdf. Accessed 18 July 2018.

Foucault, Michel. "Right of Death and Power over Life." *The Foucault Reader*, edited by Paul Rabinow, Pantheon Books, 1984, pp. 258-72.

Ford, Dana. "Attorneys: Fetus of Pregnant, Brain-Dead Wife is 'Distinctly Abnormal.'" *CNN*, 23 Jan. 2014, www.cnn.com/ 2014 /01/22/us/pregnant-life-support-texas/index.html. Accessed 18 July 2018.

Greene, Megan, and Leslie R Wolfe. "Pregnancy Exclusions in State Living Will and Medical Proxy Statutes." *Reproductive Laws for the 21st Century Papers*. Center for Women Policy Studies, 2012, np.

Gregorian, Alexis. "Post-Mortem Pregnancy: A Proposed Methodology." *Annals of Health Law*, vol. 19, no. 2, 2010, pp. 401-24.

Grosz, Elizabeth. *Space, Time, and Perversion: Essays on the Politics of Bodies*. Routledge, 1995.

Holloway, Karla FC. *Private Bodies, Public Texts*. Duke University Press, 2011.

In re Quinlan. 70 NJ 10. Supreme Court of New Jersey. *Justia U.S. Law*, 1976, law.justia.com/cases/new-jersey/supreme-court/1976/70-n-j-10-0.html. Accessed 18 July 2018.

Lederman, Anne D. "A Womb of My Own: A Moral Evaluation of Ohio's Treatment of Pregnant Patients with Living Wills." *Case Western Reserve Law Review*, vol. 45, 1994, pp. 351-77.

Miles, Stephen H, and Alison August. "Courts, Gender, and the 'Right to Die.'" *Law, Medicine, and Health Care*, vol. 18, 1990, pp. 85-95.

Munoz v. John Peter Smith Hospital. No. 096-270080-14. District Court 96th Judicial District, Tarrant County, 2014, ThaddeusPope, www.thaddeuspope.com/images/MUNOZ_-_Stipulation_Facts.pdf/. Accessed 18 July 2018.

Roe v. Wade. 410 US 113. Supreme Court of the United States. *Justia US Supreme Court*, 1973, supreme.justia.com/cases/federal/us/410/113/ Accessed 18 July 2018.

Schindler v. Schiavo. No.866 So. 2d 140. Supreme Court of the United States. *Justia US Law*, 2005, https://law.justia.com/cases/florida/second-district-court-of-appeal/2005/2d05-968.html Accessed 18 July 2018.

Sisti, Emma. "Die Free or Live: The Constitutionality of New Hampshire's Living Will Pregnancy Exception." *Vermont Law Review*, vol. 30, no. 1, 2005, pp. 143-78.

Taylor, Katherine. "Compelling Pregnancy at Death's Door." *Columbia Journal of Gender and the Law*, vol. 7, no. 1, 1997, pp. 85-165.

Health and Safety Code Section Advance Directives Act 2015. 166.001-166.209. *Government of Texas*, 2015, statutes.capitol.texas.gov/Docs/HS/htm/HS.166.htm. Accessed 18 July 2018.

Fiore, Robin. "Framing Terri Schiavo: Gender, Disability, and Fetal Protection." *The Case of Terri Schiavo: Ethics, Politics and Death in the 21st Century*, edited by Kenneth W. Goodman, Oxford University Press, 2010, pp. 191-209.

University Health Services, Inc v. Robert Piazzi. No CV86-RCCV-464. Superior Court of Richmond County. *ThaddeusPope*, 1986, www.thaddeuspope.com/images/Univrsity_Health_v_Piazzi_Ga_Sup_1986_.pdf. Accessed 18 July 2018.

Walen, Alec. "Constitutionality of States Extending Personhood to the Unborn." *Constitutional Commentary*, vol. 22, no. 1, 2012, pp. 161-80.

Chapter Four

Manufacturing the Mother: Technical Appropriations of Birth in Ancient Greek Thought

Jessica Elbert Decker

The colonization of women's bodies has a long history in Western patriarchal culture. As Jane Caputi has succinctly expressed, the "control of women's sexual and reproductive capacities is the core patriarchal practice" (392). To the Ancient Greek imagination, the maternal body was a site marked by chaos, excess, and the unruly forces of chance. This site was associated with nature itself (or herself) as fertility, corporeality, and mortality—essentially, for the Ancient Greek patriarchal imagination, women represented the keys to life and death.[1] Feminist scholars such as Nicole Loraux and Froma Zeitlin have argued that the female power of generation (birth) was repeatedly appropriated in Greek myth through narratives of male mastery. The Athenian belief in autochthony, in which men are born from the ground rather than the womb, Zeus's fantastical birth of Athena, and the creation of Pandora are all mythical examples of this appropriation. As Loraux has remarked, this dispossession of women's reproductive function "belongs to the realm of the imaginary, and it looks like the expression of a dream or a denial of reality rather than a definite program or an Athenian theory of reproduction" (9). The fantasy of parthenogenesis distances men from the chaos of the womb and fulfills a wish for not only bodily autonomy but for immortality—birth and death are symbolically linked, and before Pandora's arrival, men did not suffer or die.[2]

This appropriation of female generative power takes a very specific form, as I shall demonstrate here: mastery of nature through the practice of "*techne*." The use of *techne*— which for the Ancient Greeks meant any process of creation beginning with intelligent *conception*— is in imitation of nature but vaunted as superior to the vagaries of natural forces. The Ancient Greek concept of *techne* parallels natural reproduction with one crucial difference: whereas nature is viewed as uncanny and chaotic, the production guided by *techne* is directed by an intelligent mastery.

Mastery, control, and domination are overarching paradigms of Western patriarchy—all that threatens to exceed control, such as the exigencies of nature and the seemingly chaotic forces of the body, is projected onto an image of woman. The maternal body, perceived by the male imaginary as bringer of life and bridge between worlds, becomes the crucial battleground for patriarchal mastery.[3] The justification (which is in reality a fantastical pretense) for the domination of women's bodies is the imaginary construction of female sexuality as dangerous, excessive, and chaotic. Technical mastery has been, in Western patriarchy, the means by which this control over nature and, by extension, female bodies has been wielded. Technology has been practised according to this patriarchal paradigm of mastery with violent and destructive effects—most notably the degradation of the environment, the construction of vast weaponry, rampant sexual violence against women, and micromanagement of women's bodies that strips them of reproductive and bodily autonomy.[4]

This project is indebted to the methodology of Luce Irigaray, who suggests the structure of what Lacan called the "symbolic" is not immutable and stable, but receptive to intervention and transformation. Myth, as a direct expression of a culture's unconscious symbolic arrangements, offers a glimpse of these subterranean constellations. To excavate these hidden associations and reveal their oppressive effects, critical feminist interventions into mythological structures are necessary—especially when those structures are reflected in philosophical or scientific narratives claiming objectivity. As Donna Haraway has argued, "one important route for reconstructing socialist-feminist politics is through theory and practice addressed to the social relations of science and technology, including crucially the systems of myth and meanings structuring our imaginations" (163). Female sexuality is persistently characterized in Greek myth as dangerous, deceitful, ambiguous, and excessive. Pandora and Aphrodite, as well as her equally destructive mortal avatar Helen, are emblematic of this depiction, which is not a true account of women's so-called nature, but a male fantasy suggesting intense fears of powerlessness coupled with resentment at our animal dependence on the earth. Without making these fantasies visible, their constructions are mistaken for an immutable order of reality—which is precisely the aim of Zeus's reign in Greek myth—and a common strategy of patriarchal thought in constructing femininity as essence.

Although the mythological images of female bodies are obviously products of the cultural imagination of the time, the philosophical works of Plato and Aristotle repeat these images and enshrine them in the guise of objectivity and reason. *Techne* requires intelligent conception, and is imagined to be superior to natural creation. This belief precisely parallels an argument in Plato's *Symposium*, in which female mouthpiece Diotima emphasizes the superiority of giving birth to beautiful ideas (as men do, with their souls) over chasing immortality through the birth of children (where women and the body must be involved). The processes of nature are subject to forces of chance; *techne* is used as a strategy for escaping the whims of unpredictable nature by imposing human wishes onto it. As Aristotle tells us in the *Physics*, "*techne* either completes the work that nature is unable to complete or imitates nature" (II, 8). In this study, I hope to reveal the structure of this symbolic constellation in the patriarchal imaginary, and to establish that the contemporary obsession with managing and regulating female bodies, especially in their sexual and reproductive capacities, has deep unconscious and cultural roots. Making these structures visible is especially urgent when the patriarchal practice of *techne* expresses itself in violent fantasies and forms, such as the lust for weaponry and war.

Motherless Daughters and Weapons of War

Three familiar examples from myth will illustrate a pattern in the male imaginary: the Athenian legend of autochthony, Zeus's parthenogenic birth of Athena, and his creation of Pandora. Each of these stories is a narrative detailing the male appropriation of birth, and the stories share a significant common ingredient: the blacksmith god Hephaestus, who is associated with technical mastery and the construction of wondrous devices and weapons. Hephaestus split open Zeus's head, facilitating the birth of Athena. Hephaestus also built Pandora at Zeus's command. The Athenian belief in autochthony stems from the myth of Erichthonios—and he was born from Hephaestus's seed, when it fell onto the earth (Gaia) after Hephaestus attempted to rape the virgin goddess Athena. As Loraux argues, "Hephaistos seems predisposed to intervene in all generation that occurs without sexual reproduction" (128). The erasure of the maternal body is represented in fantasy, in these narratives, by images that include technical mastery, autonomous male creation, sexual violence, and weaponry—a constellation of images still alarmingly present in the violent ends of current Western patriarchy. After examining these three mythical examples in turn, I will suggest Plato's and Aristotle's conceptual treatments of the maternal body follow the same fantastical logic and imagery as that expressed in these tales from the Ancient Greek mythological imagination.

The feminist scholarship on the deep misogyny in Ancient Greek patriarchal culture is voluminous, so I will sketch a specific symbolic matrix for the purposes of this study. The maternal body and female sexuality more generally are marked—throughout Ancient Greek myth, religion, and cultural practice—as excessive, chaotic, dangerous, and irrational. As Froma Zeitlin has demonstrated in her work, "to isolate and insulate female *eros*, from society and from itself, was demonstrably the strategy informing many of the notions, conventions, and rituals that surrounded female life in the ancient world" (136). The physical body itself was understood as demonic and unruly: the body is an ambiguous thing: not only an intelligible object of technical mastery but also a site of strange, unruly forces" (Holmes 190). This need for mastery over the demonic physical body is especially evident in Plato, whose dualism places superior value in the soul while vilifying the body, especially for the body's excess and lack of restraint.[5] Plato's commitment to dualism can frequently be read as an attempt to quarantine male identity from contaminants, such as the animal-like body, associated with women and with ephemeral mortality.

Ancient Greek women's nature was often compared to that of animals. Cristiana Franco's recent study explores the identification of femininity as doglike; both women and dogs are identified as "shameless" and requiring male dominance. As Franco explains, shamelessness "literally means lack of *aidos*, that is, lack of restraint, the moral curb responsible for inhibiting any behavior subject to ethical censure" (9). This is particularly relevant in our reading of Pandora, who is endowed with, in Elissa Marder's clever translation, a "bitchlike" mind (13). Franco argues that the domination of women is justified by their allegedly natural excess: "the founding justification for this subordination was therefore entrusted to a cultural strategy that made both women and dogs into figures of natural excess, overflowing, intrusive, constitutionally lacking restraint, and for this reason needing corrections and restrictions of every sort" (128). With these observations in mind, the three examples examined here may be read as political strategies undergirding the desires of the patriarchal imagination—specifically the violent wish for dominance and mastery over the power of birth.

In *The Children of Athena: Athenian Ideas about Citizenship and the Division Between the Sexes*, Nicole Loraux examines the Athenian belief in autochthony, in which men are born not from the wombs of women but from the earth. Loraux suggests the following: "the doctrine of autochthony is something like the satisfaction of a desire, rather than a misunderstanding of the laws of reproduction. The desire of a society of men to deny the reality of reproduction is vested in the story of Erichthonios, since masculine experience dictates that what really counts takes place among men" (17). Rather than accept the dangerous origin of the womb, the fantasy of autochthony frees men from their umbilical bonds and offers them imaginary autonomy. Erichthonios is born when Hephaestus attempts to rape Athena; although he fails, his seed lands on her leg, and she wipes it to the ground in disgust. The resulting child, thus, has three parents: Hephaestus the father, Gaia the mother, and Athena, who fosters the child and raises him. Loraux contends that Athena represents all three of the traditional roles in the parenting of Erichthonios: she is father, mother, and nurse (*trophos*) because "she lies beyond the opposition between masculine and feminine" and she "achieves the masculine dream of the Greeks—to have a child outside the limits of procreative activity" (64). Athena is the perfect daughter of patriarchy because she is insulated from any maternal genealogies. She has no mother (the inaccessible Metis), no progeny, and no lovers. The grave danger of female sexuality, with its proximity to birth and death, is eliminated.

The story of Athena's birth begins when Zeus swallows his first wife Metis to avoid being usurped by his progeny. Metis is the goddess of cunning resourcefulness, and she is pregnant with Athena at the time of her consumption. She now guides Zeus as an internal strategist from inside of him—no longer an autonomous goddess but a permanent captive. In their extensive study of the Ancient Greek concept of *metis*, Marcel Detienne and Jean-Pierre Vernant consider the motivations and consequences of Zeus's act: "Zeus at one stroke eliminated the element of unpredictability and disorder which had previously given rise to revolts and conflicts among the gods. He replaced it with an order which was immutable" (305). Ingesting his powerful wife was, thus, a political strategy, a way of ensuring Zeus's sovereignty. The act insulates him from the vagaries of chance: "Nothing can surprise him, cheat his vigilance or frustrate his designs" (Detienne and Vernant 14). This lust for total access, for Zeuslike omniscience, is a primary impulse of Western patriarchal domination, and is represented as the antidote for chaos and disorder.[6] However, substituting the maternal body with male technicity has its violent drawbacks, even in fantasy; for Athena to be born, Hephaestus had to split open Zeus's head with a deadly weapon.

The cunning resourcefulness of Metis's maternal body is transferred to Zeus by his ingestion, and the product of his pregnancy, Athena, is, thus, a motherless male fantasy. Athena, the virgin goddess of war, is the perfect daughter of patriarchy—which is demonstrated by her function as aid to male heroes, such as Odysseus and Perseus, and her exoneration of Orestes after he murdered his mother, Clytemnestra. The virginal, warrior goddess Athena is not a danger to men; she does not seduce, trap, or usurp them. She is an image of femininity sanitized of all its threatening aspects, including the threat of chaos that her mother Metis posed. As Detienne and Vernant remark on Athena's birth: "she herself, as the goddess who emerged fully armed from

Zeus's skull, is the product of a metallurgical operation. Her blazing gaze is not the evil-eye cast by the artisan but rather the terrifying flashing of bronze which has been wrought for warlike purposes" (183). As a virgin with no progeny, Athena's body is not productive; the dangerous liminality of the maternal body is exorcised and replaced with a sleek, metal model without leaks. Neither a maternal body subject to the whims of nature nor a seductive body that could ensnare, Athena is a sharp and controlled weapon, ever poised for war at the wishes of men.

Nonetheless, Athena retains some of her forgotten mother's traits, as she represents "skill and technical inventiveness" in the Ancient Greek imagination (Detienne and Vernant 178). As the narratives reveal, she is strongly linked with Hephaestus: he is midwife to her birth, they are co-parents of Erichthonios, and she is renowned for her use of weapons forged by the blacksmith god. David Leitao also suggests that the birth of Athena "becomes a myth of cultural progress, an account of how *techne* first came into existence" (110). In other mythical narratives, Athena is consistently linked with *techne* and the appropriation of female generativity. She helps the hero Perseus to decapitate Medusa, a powerful and uncastrated female figure, and she presides over the creation of Pandora, the dangerous artifice built by Zeus and Hephaestus.[7] As Loraux writes, "there is a more subtle resemblance that links her [Athena] to the 'beautiful evil' [Pandora] conceived by Zeus: she, like the first woman, is the offspring of Zeus alone, joined to him by an exclusive bond. Indeed, the 'artificial goddess' watches over the making of the 'femme fatale' in Hesiod's poetic work" (80). Athena also famously presides over the domestication of animals—a technical taming linking her to Prometheus, whose theft of fire inspired Zeus to create Pandora.[8]

Hesiod's narratives of Pandora's creation have been the subject of many feminist analyses; for the purposes of this project—linking the appropriation of female generativity with male mastery through *techne*—the suggestions of Nicole Loraux and Elissa Marder are crucial. Zeus orders Hephaestus, the magician blacksmith god who forges weapons, to create Pandora as a punishment for Prometheus's theft of fire. Before Pandora, men lived in a kind of utopian state, a world without women, suffering, or toil. To mitigate the godlike power that men would wield through the use of fire, Zeus puts them back in their place by creating the race of women. In Hesiod's *Works and Days*, Zeus proclaims that Pandora is "an evil in which they all may rejoice in spirit as they embrace their own destruction" (57-59). The theme of *techne* in this myth not only appears in the creation of the artifice Pandora, but is also implicated in the events leading up to her creation, as fire is an emblematic symbol of *techne*. (Hephaestus the blacksmith god cannot create his weapons or devices without fire.)

Loraux was the first to remark upon the artificial nature of Pandora: "woman, then, is an artificial creation representing the union of Zeus' conceptual project and the technical skill of Hephaistos, the artisan" (79). Loraux demonstrates that rather than linking women with birth, Pandora "takes us far from the reproductive woman" (74). Marder picks up Loraux's argument and remarks that Pandora's nature is such that "in today's parlance, we might call her an android, a robot, or a replicant" (9). As a technological image of the first woman, Pandora comes with a dangerous accessory—her famous "box" or jar (*pithos*) from which all the evils of the world emerge. The denigration of the female body, the womb in particular, is blatantly obvious in this narrative. In reading the meaning of Pandora's box, scholars generally remark on its relation to the womb; however, Marder argues that just as Pandora is not a natural mother but a fabricated object, the jar can be understood as "a *mechanical reproduction* of the womb rather than as a *representation* of it" (16, emphasis in original). The myth is ambiguous as to how Pandora creates the race of women—does she give birth to them or do they also emerge from the jar? Can she give birth if she is a technological creation of Zeus and she was never born herself? Thus, the distinction between natural reproduction (birth) and technological creation is radically obscured by this tale.

Through the creation of Pandora, the maternal body as origin of life is effaced, and birth becomes a technical male achievement. Even the context for this creation exhibits patriarchal patterns: Pandora is created to settle the score between two warring males, Zeus and Prometheus. Marder's reading of this narrative, as it is told in Hesiod's *Theogony* and his *Works and Days*, demonstrates that "the concept of 'the mother' has always been paradoxical and that the idea of human birth has always already been marked by *technological* figures, fears, desires, anxieties" (9, emphasis in original). As Rosi Braidotti has noted, this is not an isolated case, but reflects a pattern—there is "intense uterus envy built into technological culture" (208). The same symbolic patterns enumerated here appear, in startling detail, in the philosophical texts of both Plato and Aristotle.

Imagination Becomes Institution: Plato and Aristotle

A thorough investigation of the maternal body in Plato and Aristotle would be an immense undertaking; for the purposes of this analysis, I would like to gesture toward a few of their key texts and sketch, in broad strokes, the parallels between their philosophical systems and the mythological patterns outlined above. In Plato, the metaphor of pregnancy in *Symposium* and the demiurge creating the cosmos in *Timaeus* will be the points of focus. Diotima's speech in *Symposium* suggests that the female power of birth is inferior to male pregnancy of soul, in which men give birth to beautiful ideas instead of children. In the *Timaeus*, the figure of the demiurge introduces male technical mastery into a cosmology that, tellingly, relies on the model of the reproductive family—father, mother, and child—in outlining the origin of the cosmos. In the case of Aristotle, my exposition relies on Emanuela Bianchi's reading of technicity as a theme in *Generation of Animals*, in which Aristotle details the processes of sexual reproduction.

In the *Symposium*, Plato's dialogue about love, prominent Athenian men take turns making speeches to the god Eros. Phaedrus, the first speaker, takes a quote from Parmenides out of context—"she contrived *eros* first of all the gods"—and argues that Eros is the oldest of the gods, when he is, in fact, the child of the goddess Aphrodite (the "she" of the quotation).[9] This "program of suppressing the mother" in the dialogue, as Leitao describes it, continues in the speech of Pausanias, who divides Aphrodite into two forms—the vulgar Aphrodite (Pandemos) and the heavenly Aphrodite (Urania) in order to argue the superiority of Aphrodite Urania as motherless, born from the seed of Uranus alone (193). As Leitao argues, "Pausanias' distinction ... not only privileges the exclusive parthenogenetic creativity of the male (Uranus) over the sexual reproduction of male and female ... but also anticipates, on the level of myth, the transition from physical (Pandemus) to spiritual (Urania) procreation that we will encounter in the philosophical ascent described by Diotima" (193). Diotima begins her famous speech by offering a genealogy of the god Eros; she says he descends from his mother Penia (Poverty) and his father Poros (Resourcefulness) (203b-e). This story of the birth of Eros has no basis in mythical tradition and is strategically invented by Plato to serve his arguments.

Just as Aphrodite is replaced with the male deity Eros, here the goddess Metis is replaced with a male figure, Poros—who is supposedly the son of Metis, although she has no offspring in myth, as she was swallowed before she could give birth to Athena. The qualities Eros allegedly inherits from this father are enumerated: "a famous hunter, always weaving some stratagem; desirous and competent of wisdom, throughout life ensuing the truth; a master of jugglery, witchcraft, and artful speech" (203d). The mother of Eros is described in less glowing terms, as she conceives her son through somehow raping Poros while he is drunk and unconscious.[10] Of course, this genealogy is aimed at describing the nature of Eros as simultaneously resourceful (Poros) and in a constant state of lack (Penia), but this gendered characterization is not entirely innocent when viewed in the larger context of Plato's arguments in the *Symposium.*

The fantasy of male pregnancy is employed to demonstrate that the intelligent conception of beautiful ideas is superior to the physical conception of children. Plato is clear that this intelligent activity is the province of men, whereas he derides birth as bodily, female, and distinctly inferior.[11] Furthermore, Plato strategically places this speech in the mouth of an imaginary woman, as he attempts to drive home the point that, as Diotima herself states, "every one would choose to have got children such as these [beautiful ideas] rather than the human sort" (209d). Men are pregnant in both body and soul, and "those who are teeming in body betake them rather to women," whereas male pregnancy of soul conceives of immortal things, such as virtue and prudence (208e-209a). Thus giving birth to children is cast as a shadow or imitation of true creation; true creation is celebrated as rational, male, and *ethical.* Diotima's speech in the *Symposium* undermines the female power of birth by identifying it as a superficial (bodily) bid for immortality, and contrasts it with the exercise of male intelligence in giving birth to beautiful ideas.

Plato's *Timaeus* reveals the connection between this celebration of male conception and mastery of the physical world through *techne;* his figure of the male demiurge—called both father and poet—produces the entire cosmos through technical artistry.[12] The *Timaeus* is an unusual dialogue for various reasons, perhaps most notably because it is the only dialogue where Plato offers a cosmology. The cosmos, described as a living being, comes about through a process analogous to sexual reproduction. Plato uses the model of the family— father, mother, and child—as the structure in his explanation. Thus, the narrative Plato weaves is a story about the origin of life, and he places a male craftsman, the demiurge, behind the birth of the cosmos. As Sara Brill argues, this demiurge's activities allow for the "elision of technical production and sexual reproduction" (163). The demiurge orders the cosmos, which he finds in a state of chaos—"the world encountered by the demiurge at the beginning of the dialogue is 'discordant and disordered motion'" (Bianchi, "Receptacle/Chora" 135). He is called a poet because he is not merely the origin of life, but he is endowed with the power to weave *order* and narrative—just as Plato himself does in offering the cosmology.

The description associated with the mother falls outside of Plato's usual binary between the sensible and intelligible; he posits a "third kind" he calls "*khora.*" This strange third kind is "some invisible but shapeless form—all receptive, but partaking somehow of the intelligible in the most perplexing way" (51a-b). *Khora*—sometimes designated as receptacle, sometimes as space, sometimes as mother or nurse, and sometimes as a "molding stuff for everything" (50c)—has no real character of its own but takes the form of whatever is impressed into it.[13] "The figures that come into it and go out of it are always imitations of the things that *are,* having been imprinted from them in some manner hard to tell of and wondrous" (50c). Thus, the figure of the mother is elided and made instead into a "receptacle for all becoming, a sort of wet-nurse" (49b). Instead of figuring the mother as the origin of the cosmos, the male demiurge, as father, functions as the "wondrous" means by which forms are imprinted on the mother (*khora*). As Sara Brill remarks, "this cosmogony posits a masculine human prototype whose actions generate the need for sexually differentiated bodies, thereby enshrining masculinity as a fecund generative force in the cosmos" (162). Human beings are originally male, and only become female through the failure to live well; if the soul persists in evil, it will "take on some such bestial nature in the similitude of that mode of life that was born in him" (42c).

Once again, as in *Symposium,* the ethical character of the soul is distinctly masculine, whereas women are cast in the same amoral realm as animals. Brill comments on the effect of this explanation of sexual difference, and argues that Plato grounds "an originary masculinity of the human kind, and the emergence of sexual difference as a secondary expression of the moral status of an individual soul" (167). Similarly, Bianchi points out that the description and function of *khora* "crucially involves a relegation of the feminine to a position of barely knowable, shifting, erratic function in the production of a metaphysical system and world in which only men are able to function as fully agentic, reasoning beings" ("Receptacle/Chora" 125). The activity of the demiurge is contrasted with the activities of nature, and these are designated as two different kinds of *cause*: "on one side those which, with the aid of intellect, are craftsmen of things beautiful and good, on the other side those which, bereft of prudence, produce on each occasion a disordered, chance effect" (46e). The parallel here to the two kinds of pregnancy in *Symposium* is obvious and consistent with Plato's preference for the soul over the body (and active male over passive female).

The theme of male mastery as *techne* in Plato's figure of the demiurge is taken up by Aristotle in his narratives of sexual reproduction. Bianchi, in *The Feminine Symptom: Aleatory Matter in the Aristotelian Cosmos*, has persuasively demonstrated that Aristotle's metaphysical system is grounded in his understanding of biology. Aristotle attributes gendered functions to his concepts of matter and form: matter is passive and feminine whereas form is masculine and actively directed by intelligence. Plato's image of the male craftsman imprinting form onto the passive feminine moulding stuff of the receptacle, *khora*, is repeated in Aristotle's models of sexual reproduction. In *Generation of Animals*, Aristotle states that the principle of soul present in males is what allows them to impose form onto matter in the same way that a carpenter imposes form onto materials; he then goes on to say that sperm works in exactly this way (*kata technen*) when it imposes form on passive feminine matter in animal reproduction (I, 22:15-25). Commenting on this passage, Bianchi argues "Aristotle in this way installs a technicity, a scene of artifactual production, at the heart of natural generation, which is thereby ineluctably marked as an operation of the masculine upon the feminine, the active upon the passive" (*Symptom* 2). The role of the mother in reproduction is merely that of receptacle and material;

she cannot contribute to the creation of the child's soul, and, instead, her only effect on generation is that of distortion.

In *Timaeus*, the demiurge, described as perfectly good, "willed that all things should come to resemble himself as much as possible" (29e). This fantasy of autonomous creation is echoed in Aristotle's narrative of sexual reproduction, as is Plato's suggestion that maleness is the original form, whereas femaleness is a kind of accident or contingency.[14] Just as resemblance was the basis for the demiurge's activity of creation in forming things that resemble himself, the child begotten by the father, in Aristotle's model, would resemble the father exactly were it not for the distorting influence of the mother's chaotic body. Thus, when a female child is born, it is paradoxically in accordance with nature (since, after all, females are needed for reproduction to occur) and simultaneously accidental. Bianchi points out the significant language associated with Aristotle's explanation: in the creation of a female child, "nature *strays* from kind, and the male fails to 'gain the mastery' (*kratein* is a concept familiar from political contexts, carrying the sense of seizing control and ruling that may also be understood as an establishment of sovereignty)" (*Symptom* 38, emphasis in original). This political language of mastery is no accident; the metaphysical systems of Plato and Aristotle repeat, in symbolic form, the strategies of Zeus in his struggle to maintain the patriarchal cosmos.

Although the symbolic constellation outlined here reveals that *techne* has been practised in accordance with the patriarchal paradigms of mastery and dominance, this is not to suggest that technology takes this form of necessity—revealing the contingency of its character in Western patriarchal society is the first step in exploring new paths for technological practice. The elision of the maternal body in Ancient Greek thought not only contributes to the concrete oppression of women in patriarchal society but tends to set the practice of *techne* against nature—*techne* becomes a means of *conquering* nature and is, thus, a force opposed to life, in its many prolific forms. Combined with the Zeuslike desire for total control, *techne* becomes a weapon, an instrument of war; nature (of which the maternal body is emblematic) becomes the enemy that must be vanquished. In the symbolic constellations explored in this analysis, female bodies—especially that of the mother—are denied agency and categorized as manifestations of chaotic, irrational nature, whereas only men are capable of creation through *techne*. These patterns in the patriarchal male imaginary do not merely appear in the colourful myths of the Ancient Greek world, but quietly slip into philosophical and scientific discourses that claim objectivity, like those of Plato and Aristotle. While the fantastical nature of these symbolic arrangements remains invisible, the agency of female bodies will continue to be undermined, and the female power of birth will continue to be managed through male paradigms of mastery. Until the patriarchal practice of *techne* as mastery and domination is critically examined and effectively sabotaged by feminist interventions, its destructive effects will continue: in the degradation of the environment, in the lust for limitless weaponry, and in the constant domination over women's bodies, especially in their reproductive capacities.

Endnotes

1 See Jean-Pierre Vernant's "Feminine Faces of Death" for a detailed discussion of the manner in which women are associated with death in Ancient Greek myth and culture.

2 The fantasy of parthenogenesis is not limited to Ancient Greek myth, but also appears in psychoanalytic theory; see "The Medusa Complex: Matricide and the Fantasy of Castration" (Mayock) for analysis of parthenogenesis as a core fantasy of Western patriarchy.

3 By "male imaginary," I mean to indicate the symbolic realm of myth and culture, which, in the Ancient Greek world, and in our contemporary patriarchy, is male dominated.

4 The Ancient Greek concept of techne is broader than our contemporary category of technology, as techne included art, poetry, and craftsmanship, although the practice of both techne and technology invoke the paradigm of intelligent mastery.

5 It is important to note that mind-body dualism was not prevalent in the poetic and philosophical tradition that preceded Plato (Homer, Hesiod, and pre-Socratic thinkers).

6 This need for total visibility as fantasized control is disturbingly evident in the contemporary patriarchal structures of the panoptic surveillance state and in seemingly innocuous medical imaging practices such as the ultrasound.

7 For analysis of Medusa as an uncastrated and powerful woman (Freud's "phallic mother"), see Mayock "The Medusa Complex: Matricide and the Fantasy of Castration."

8 Franco points out that both Athena and Prometheus are skillful in the domestication of animals. She also notes that some of Athena's epithets reveal this designation as well, such as Athena "Oxbinder" (43).

9 Parmenides, DK28b13; cited in the speech of Phaedrus, in *Symposium* 178b.

10 "Now Poros, grown tipsy with nectar—for wine as yet there was none—went into the garden of Zeus, and there, overcome with heaviness, slept. Then Penia, being of herself so resourceless devised the scheme of having a child by Poros, and lying down by his side she conceived Eros" (203b-c).

11 It is also worth noting that throughout Diotima's discussion, female pregnancy and male siring of children are equated, further eliding the role of the maternal body.

12 It is significant, given the patterns outlined here, that the *Timaeus* is said to take place during the Panathenaea, a festival celebrating Athena as divine patroness of Athens.

13 The Ancient Greek word for "molding stuff" is "*ekmageion*"; Emanuela Bianchi analyzes this concept in depth in *The Feminine Symptom: Aleatory Matter in the Aristotelian Cosmos*, pages, 90-94. She emphasizes the influence of Plato's khora on Aristotle's conceptions of aleatory matter (consistently described as feminine).

14 Bianchi's focus on what she calls the feminine symptom takes up this language of a fall; "*sumptoma* is literally a falling together ... anything that befalls one, a chance, mischance, or calamity" (*Symptom* 7).

Works Cited

Aristotle. *Generation of Animals*. Translated by A.L. Peck, Harvard University Press, 1942.

Aristotle. *Physics*. Translated by Terrence Irwin Gail Fine, Hackett Publishing Company, 1995.

Bianchi, Emanuela. *The Feminine Symptom: Aleatory Matter in the Aristotelian Cosmos*. Fordham University Press, 2014. Print.

Bianchi, Emanuela. "Receptacle/Chora: Figuring the Errant Feminine in Plato's *Timaeus.*" *Hypatia*, vol. 21, no. 4, 2006, pp. 124-46.

Braidotti, Rosi. *Metamorphoses: Towards a Materialist Theory of Becoming.* Blackwell Publishers, 2002.

Caputi, Jane. *Goddesses and Monsters: Women, Myth, Power, and Popular Culture.* University of Wisconsin Press, 2004.

Detienne, Marcel, and Jean-Pierre Vernant. *Cunning Intelligence in Greek Culture and Society.* University of Chicago Press, 1991.

Franco, Cristiana. *Shameless: The Canine and the Feminine in Ancient Greece.* University of California Press, 2014.

Haraway, Donna Jeanne. *Simians, Cyborgs, and Women: The Reinvention of Nature.* Routledge, 1991.

Hesiod. *Works and Days.* Loeb Classical Library, Harvard University Press, 2006.

Holmes, Brooke. *The Symptom and the Subject.* Princeton University Press, 2010.

Leitao, David. *The Pregnant Male in Myth and Metaphor in Classical Greek Literature.* Cambridge University Press, 2012.

Loraux, Nicole. *The Children of Athena: Athenian Ideas About Citizenship and the Division Between the Sexes.* Princeton University Press, 1993.

Marder, Elissa. *The Mother in the Age of Mechanical Reproduction.* Fordham University Press, 2012.

Mayock, Jessica Elbert. "The Medusa Complex: Matricide and the Fantasy of Castration." *philoSOPHIA: A Journal for Continental Feminism*, vol. 3, no. 2, 2013, pp. 158-74.

Plato. *Symposium.* Translated by W. R. M. Lamb, Harvard University Press, 1925.

Plato. *Timaeus.* Translated by R.G. Bury, Harvard University Press, 1929.

Vernant, Jean-Pierre. "Feminine Faces of Death." *Mortals and Immortals*, edited by Froma Zeitlin. Princeton University Press, 199, pp. 95-110.

Zeitlin, Froma, David Halperin, and John Winkler, editors. *Before Sexuality: The Construction of Erotic Experience in the Greek World.* Princeton University Press, 1990.

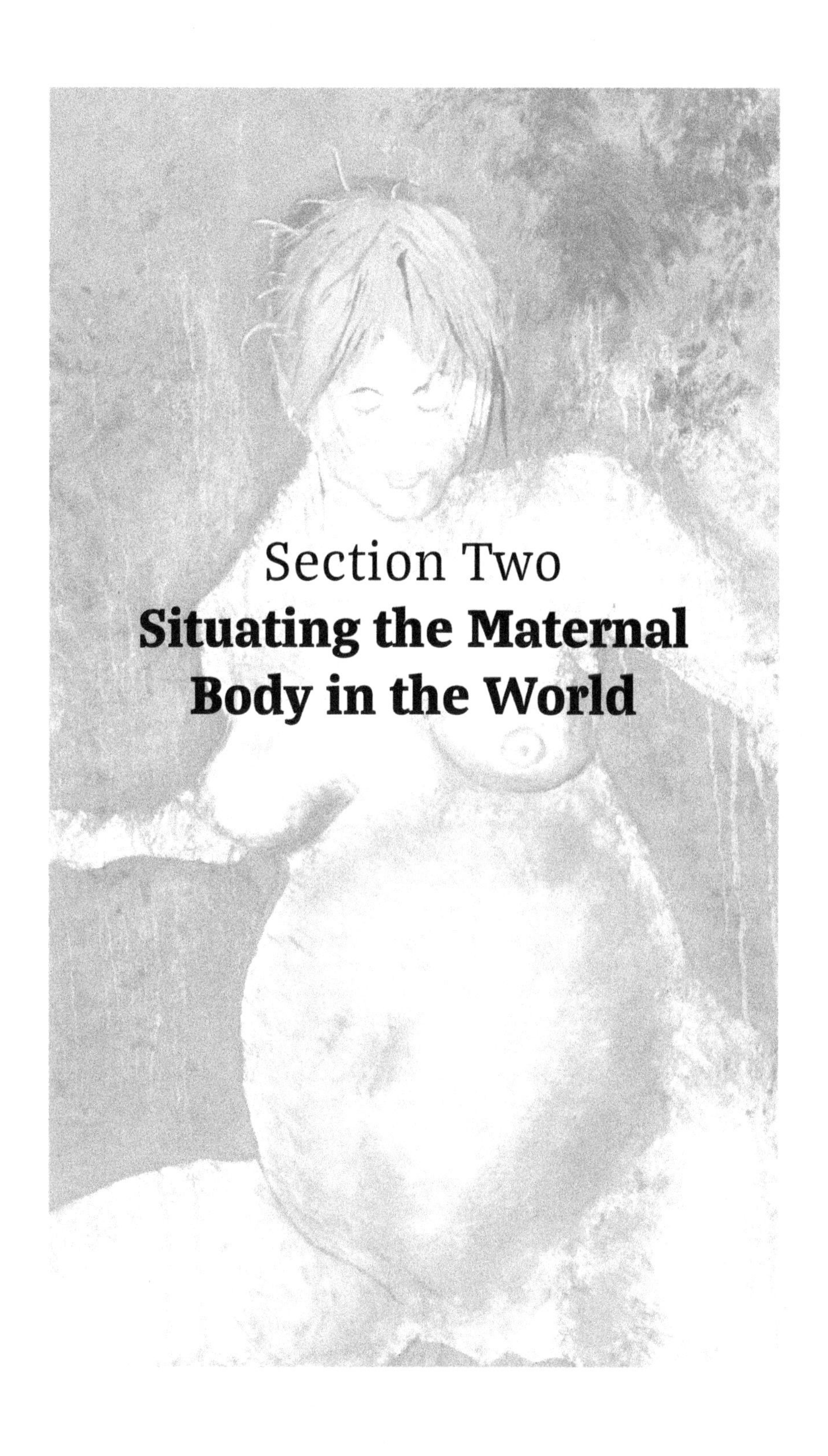

Section Two
Situating the Maternal Body in the World

Chapter Five

Seeding the Future: Maternal Microbiome as Maternal Embodiment

Rebecca Howes-Mischel

"The Maternal Microbiome: Moms Bombard Their Babies with Bugs Both Before and After They're Born" (Grens).

Grens's alliterative title and lede for the online popular science magazine *The Scientist*, stated above, reflects a push to translate suggestive findings of research on human health outcomes into content for lay audiences. In this case, Grens's post presents data from a research article released the same day in the academic journal *Science Translational Medicine* (Aagaard et al.) about newly understood symbiotic relations between maternal and fetal bodies: not only are maternal environments not as sterile as once thought, but fetal and child health seem to be influenced by exposure to multiple microbial environments throughout gestation. Although Grens's description of these findings seems at first seemingly counterintuitive—isn't one of the key features of modern mothering practices the isolation of children (particularly newborns) from unhygienic encounters?—this research is part of a growing (if contested) scientific consensus about the importance of human microbiomes. Such research argues that these diverse colonies of bacteria, fungi, and other microbes found throughout our bodies are central to understanding not only health and disease but also the development of both individual and population-level outcomes. Framing the human body as a series of interrelated ecosystems, the research Grens reviews reformulates maternal-fetal bodily relations in terms of intergenerational microbial exchanges (mediated by the placenta, vagina, and breast).

Grens's post is illustrative of a broader phenomenon in which emergent research at the intersections of microbiology and public health is transformed into public consciousness—research potentially challenging extant notions by upending some, and reaffirming other, longstanding expectations about how the maternal body is implicated in fetal and child development. Furthermore, this post reflects a current trend of simultaneously publishing technical academic articles and accessible popular science ones, which filter cutting-edge scientific findings immediately into public conversation. Although the original scientific research continues to be largely descriptive and circumspect, public writing about such research—tasked with translating its import out of the lab and into bodies—often makes broader and largely promissory claims. Attending to such transformations from academic to popular science writing, thus, offers a window into the ways new scientific claims are made socially meaningful as they are placed within existing narratives about bodily relations. Thus, even though the idea that "moms bombard their babies with bugs" (as a good thing!) is novel, it resonates within longstanding constructions of maternal bodies as materially consequential. From Aristotelian models of the body that understood maternal contribution to fetal development as merely the "soil" in which paternal seed germinated, to postgenomic life sciences that frame the maternal body as an environment contributing to future life course (Lappé; Richardson)—scholars have long positioned pregnant embodiment as determinative of future life-course development.

I argue that the maternal body emerging in human microbiome research is both material and materializing. Drawing on a feminist materialist framework (Pitts-Taylor), such analysis examines how scientific research and writing constructs its own objects; that is, how social constructs (in this case, entrenched ideas about maternal embodiment) shape biological materiality itself (in this case, the maternal microbiome). In this schema the maternal body is material: it is a fleshy and interactive microbial ecosystem reflecting an individual person's life context, which serves as a bounded environment for fetal development. And the maternal microbiome is materializing: not only does the maternal body nourish the growing fetus, but its microbiome "seeds" child life-course development through intergenerational "bug bombardment." Through critical discourse analysis of translational and public science writing about gendered microbiomes, this chapter explores the implications of such narratives that frame maternal bodies as newly consequential for fetal-child development. In particular, I argue that public representations of the maternal microbiome as a form of gendered embodiment echo longstanding narratives about the maternal body as symbolic and material terrain of future health and harm. These narratives ultimately raise questions about how pregnant people's embodiment is publicly scrutinized. Moreover, they reproduce social expectations conflating the physical and relational practices of mothering such that pregnancy itself is framed anew as form of embodied and interpersonal nurturing.

Data for this article are drawn from a multiyear analysis of peer-reviewed scientific, news reporting, and popular media about vaginal microbiomes; since 2014, I have been tracking basic research and media reports about such research alongside what could be considered "populist research," through which a sexed (and implicitly raced) human emerges as a series of microbiotic relationships. I present a close reading of reporting about the maternal microbiome and its relationship to future infant-child susceptibility to asthma, allergies, and metabolic conditions, the so-called conditions of modernity. My analysis focuses on what Emily Martin terms "the sleeping metaphors of science" ("The Egg and Sperm" 501) through which research is made socially legible to illustrate how public incorporation of new research relies on and reproduces existing social discourses about maternal embodiment. To situate this analysis, I first consider how moms matter in academic and lay articles focused on maternal bodies as environments shaping individual life course and health outcomes. In particular, I place new clinical applications of microbiome research in the context of extant anxieties about the biomedicalization of birth and of global epidemiological trends toward increasing rates of Caesarean births. I then turn to the way such scholarship on the influence of individual maternal embodiment is scaled up to explain population level health transitions in the award-winning science documentary *Microbirth.*

These examples are not meant to be exhaustive. I do not survey the full range of research on human microbiomes, which is beyond the scope of this chapter. Instead, I selected examples on the basis of what has been particularly well covered in popular science reporting—those influencing public consciousness about maternal embodiment and potentially shifting the range of ways pregnancy is felt in and through the body. Thus, though grounded in research science, this chapter analyzes popular science rhetoric to consider its public plausibility within a broader terrain of existing social, technical, and gendered politics.

The Mattering of Maternal Embodiment

Although the focus of this analysis is on emergent science writing, it is important to situate it within extant public concerns about pregnancy as a particular kind of embodied state. As Deborah Lupton notes, public discourse about the importance of the pregnant body as the locus of fetal health and harm has escalated over the last three decades. Mothering is an activity of being in relation to another, and maternal bodies have long engendered symbolic suspicion because of the way such connections render them metaphorically and materially permeable, fluid, and leaky. These bodies challenge cultural ideas that individual persons are unambiguously bounded in the skin of an individual body. Shifting registers of subjectivity, mothering as a form of embodied relationship begins prenatally as women are encouraged to think about their bodies as environments determining child outcomes; this begins even preconception as Miranda Waggoner's scholarship demonstrates. This focus on maternal bodily practices determining or alleviating risk bounds reproduction within the maternal body and return us to the Aristotelian "seed and soil theory": the seed (sperm) animates fetal life, whereas the soil (maternal body) merely gives it an environment in which to grow (Delaney). Even within current understandings of reproductive contribution in which each parent's gametes equally shape fetal life, there is stubborn attachment to the expectation that the maternal body "matters" more than the paternal one. In their analysis of the varied "reproductive equations" used to account for maternal and paternal contribution to fetal-child outcomes, Rene Almeling and Miranda Waggoner demonstrate that preconception health campaigns reiterate this view of differential contribution: "While men often receive credit for establishing a pregnancy, they are not assigned much responsibility for fetal health. As a result, preconception care researchers have to work to create a conceptual link between men's behaviour around the time of conception and pregnancy outcomes" (829). Much as Martin shows in *Woman in the Body*—wherein medical models of reproduction render the gendered body in machinelike terms and attribute labour to uterus as agent and woman as individual— contemporary prenatal and preconception campaigns focus on social and environmental risks to fetal outcomes rather than to the pregnant body, while still holding the latter responsible for the former (Lupton; McNaughton; Weir)

As Monica Casper argues, developments in biomedical and scientific understanding and treatment of fetuses as separable individuals with identifiable best interests in the 1980s and 1990s enabled an expansion of mothering responsibility from postnatal caregiving practices to prenatal caregiving behaviours. Medical and political institutions could now separate fetal bodies from maternal bodies and treat them as autonomous from maternal bodily experience. Early public health campaigns focusing on pregnant women's alcohol (Armstrong) and tobacco (Oaks) use as forms of abuse popularized this expectation that maternal embodiment was a form of responsible caregiving: "Framing pregnancy as a potential conflict (in which a woman's rights, needs, or desires clash with those of her fetus) has opened the so-called maternal-fetal relationship to public surveillance, regulation, and intervention" (Oaks 64). States have used such an understanding of the perilousness of maternal bodies to incarcerate women for prenatal drug use using expanded definitions of child abuse (Beckett). New understandings of fetal care positioned women as more or less responsible mothers on the basis of the way their bodily state may influence fetal development.

As Elizabeth Armstrong's research demonstrates, these public health campaigns took circumspect science and translated it into blanket warnings. For example, there is little research on the way varied amounts of alcohol consumed by people with different bodily histories at different points in pregnancy influences fetal development, yet American public health associations argue that pregnant women should consume zero alcohol. As activities such as maternal drinking and smoking were rendered pathological, pregnant women were tasked with experiencing pregnancy as a practice of embodying a good fetal environment. Notably, even as researchers increasingly take environmental, social, and behavioural context into account to explain determinates of fetal outcomes, their analyses of such contexts are bounded by the maternal body. As Cynthia Daniels argues, although paternal contribution is increasingly established as consequential to fetal development, it is still underaddressed by public health campaigns as a consequence of the "social construction of procreation," such that "the link between fathers and fetuses must always pass through the female body" (581). Even as fetal outcomes research considers the impact of social, environmental, and structural contexts, women are still largely held responsible for producing good outcomes, and their bodies bear the weight of such responsibility.

Postgenomic life sciences research—into which microbiome research falls—marks a further turn away from single-determinate models of life course outcomes given its focus on bodily relations as contextual, contextualizing, fluid, and interpenetrating (Lappé and Landecker). Such research instead shifts us toward narratives about the maternal body as an "environment of consequence" (Lappé 676), which resurrects the soil metaphor while extending it temporally and molecularly. This turn toward the environment as the central metaphor to explain maternal contribution to fetal development—rather than the determinism of early genetics discourses—suggests a model for understanding material relations as dispersed and causal responsibility as distributed. This research highlights the way our bodies remember social and environmental contexts intergenerationally, the way stress is a materializing force of social policies, and the variation of individual people's embodied experiences (Lappé and Landecker). However, as Sarah Richardson's analysis of "gender and the explanatory landscape of epigenetics" demonstrates, even as epigenetics moves beyond a certain kind of determinism to explain maternal-fetal relations by highlighting the significance of biosocial environments, their conclusions ultimately uphold the bounded maternal body as the "epigenetic vector" of "social determinates of health" (221). Thus, the maternal body as a bounding context—as *the* environment—remains at the centre of such narratives about fetal outcomes. Furthermore, though less explicitly tied to surveillance politics than maternal smoking and alcohol research, public narratives about such research still implicate women's bodily status as the determining context for "conditions of modernity"—including child obesity (Maher et al.;

Warin et al.), chemical exposure (Mackendrick), and autism (Lappé). Even as emergent research pushes us toward rethinking the metaphor of the body as permeable to—and reflective of—socially and politically stratified contexts, in practice, women are still held responsible for cultivating kinds of bodily states in the name of fetal interests. Public writing about the maternal microbiome fits squarely into this discourse, which materializes the maternal body via molecular relations as a consequential, and cultivatable, terrain for child development.

Ecosystemic Body-Persons

Microbiota are central to contemporary narratives about post-genomic human disorders. The magazines *Science* and *Nature* have dedicated sections to aggregating breaking research and have published special issues focused on its translational applications; similarly, in 2015, *Scientific America* devoted a special innovations issue to the suggestive promises of microbiome research. These findings populate the science and opinion sections of the *New York Times*, the *New Yorker*, National Public Radio (NPR), and proliferate across the popular and science blogospheres. They seep into popular discourses of pregnancy care, animate conversations about birth plans, and influence how prospective parents understand the roots of childhood health and their perceived responsibilities.

Coined by Noble Laureate Joshua Lederberg in 2001, the term "microbiome" refers to the genome of collective microorganisms in a given environment, whereas the term "microbiota" refers to the taxonomy of these collective microorganisms. In their often interchangeable use, these terms articulate a simultaneously ecological and genomic concept that respatializes the human body into a series of not-fully-human ecosystems. Likening the body to an unexplored continent, Francis Collins hailed the 2012 results of the Human Microbiome Project (HMP) consortium's efforts as "like 15th century explorers describing the outline of a new continent, HMP researchers employed a new technological strategy to define, for the first time, the normal microbial makeup of the human body" (NIH). Indeed, ever increasingly, and publically, individuals are asked to conceptualize themselves from within. Public discourses about optimizing bodily health reproduce provocative statistics that encourage people to distinguish between embodying as human and embodying as nonhuman: for example, the American Academy of Microbiology estimates that the actual average human body carries around about three times more microbial cells than mammalian ones; the average human microbiome weighs about 2.5 pounds and, a single human microbiome can be made up of trillions of microbes divided into thousands of species (Reid and Green).[1] This multitude is segmented into five distinct human microbiomes: skin, mouth/throat, respiratory system, stomach and intestines (gut), and urogenital, each of which will contain different numbers and strains of microbes. Accompanying these statistics are carefully stated promises about the potential that microbiota may have to heal or prevent the modern conditions, such as obesity and arthritis, although the translational scientific community is markedly reserved about these possibilities.

Suggesting that explanatory models have moved away from the epochs of the gene and the brain, in May 2016 the Obama administration committed $121 million in public funds for fiscal years 2016 and 2017 to support the National Microbiome Initiative. Rather than centring the human as exceptional—as the Human Genome Project and BRAIN initiatives did—the National Microbiome Project's focus on both human and nonhuman microbial ecosystems reframes the body-person as an ecological context. Rendering the materiality of the human body as symbiotic terrain suggests a symbolic permeability between interior and exterior, which calls into question the quintessential boundness of the human body-person. As such, it marks a shift away from the post-Enlightenment expectation that human persons are autonomous selves bounded within essentially impermeable bodies (Mauss).

Instead, an ecosystemic model for embodiment reconfigures the materiality of the human body-person as always relational, as responsive to the people around us, and as tying us to nonhuman connections. For example, although the Human Microbiome Project's 2012 report established a standardized baseline of a normal microbial colony, subsequent research has attended to differences between racialized populations (Yatsunenko), and has emphasized the importance of environmental context across generation, especially in research comparing modern, and preindustrial or Indigenous populations (Segata). Moreover, these sources stress that microbiomes are not fixed; they change over our lifetime but even, possibly, in increments as small as a day. In science writer Ed Yong's words, "the microbiome is the sum of our experiences throughout our lives: the genes we inherited, the drugs we took, the food we ate, the hands we shook."

This presents a paradox. On the one hand, people are encouraged to cultivate a good microbiomic body through consumption of probiotic or fermented food (or even dirt), yet, on the other, they must understand their bodies as already marked by such histories. Microbiome writing, thus, treads a fine line between the contained suggestiveness of lab-based data—the complicated biosocial interpersonal contexts that are "datafied" to make claims about complex phenomena such as malnutrition—and the speculative market in aspirational commodities targeting the microbiome (Benezra). For anthropologists and other science studies researchers, efforts to represent the embodied person as ecosystemic, thus, raise intriguing questions about how to account for the material and materialization of raced, gendered, and situated humans while "transforming our categories of 'community,' 'individual,' and 'life'" (Benezra et al. 6380). This paradigm shift in the life sciences toward an ecosystemic model also suggests a retrenchment of gender as materially embodied and maternally embodied in consequential ways for understanding the conflations of maternal bodies with mothering bodies.

Although much of the initial popular media about microbiotic-selves has centred on the importance of gut ecosystems for everything from immune system strength to body size to predilection for depression, increasingly the vaginal environment is receiving clinical and public attention. Intriguingly dynamic, healthy vaginal microbiomes (defined by primarily by the absence of *bacterial vaginosis*, BV) show no uniformity in their so-called bacterial fingerprint and evince a "dynamism" appearing to be impervious to outside interference (Hickey et al.). As one recent popular science review article framed it, the vagina's resilient and self-contained nature appears as a mystery in which the same microbe might be interchangeably a "hero" or "villain" (Powell). Even though one researcher has termed vaginas a "self-cleaning oven," vaginal environments are firmly bound to and reflect broader social contexts—as women with lower educational attainment and income near or below the poverty line have higher rates of BV (Allsworth et al.). Finally, vaginal ecosystems respond to shifts in reproductive activity—reacting to unprotected sex and adapting to pregnancy (Aagaard et al., "A Metagenomics Approach").

Vaginal environments also facilitate intergenerational microbial relations, and constitute a kind of matrilineal inheritance passed from mother to child. For although placentas contain small colonies of microbes, there is growing consensus that infants' gut microbiomes are initially set (or "seeded") as they pass through the birth canal (Mueller et al.), and connect early immune system development to maternal microbial contribution. Conversely, in a medically sterile Caesarean birth, a child's initial gut colonies are seeded by the skin microbiomes of both parents (Dominguez-Bello et al., "Delivery Mode Shapes"). Correspondingly some research shows that infants born by Caesarean section and fed formula have gut microbiomes with decreased microbial population and genomic variation (Bäckhed et al.), although subsequent research may contest the strength of this finding (Stewart et al.). In this new attention to the influence of the maternal vaginal microbiome on babies' gut colonies, vaginas are cast as sites of future possibility—forms of attachment that entangle intergenerational connection, potential, and harm.

"Mom Matters"

A key question in postgenomic life sciences is how does maternal embodiment matter in establishing conditions for fetal harm and health? How can we understand maternal embodiment as linking us molecularly and temporally to and through kin, history, and environmental context—to both past and future generations? Tasking microbiomes with answering these questions shifts the questions themselves into ones about how moms "matter" in a double sense—both as literal bodily material and as consequential for the development of initial microbiome, immune, and metabolic health. As Grens sums up in *The Scientist* post that began this piece:

> the placental microbiome likely represents a baby's first meeting with the microbial world. The birthing process, then, would be the second stop on a tour of the maternal microbiome. Once on the outside, a baby's first embrace with his mother is really a group hug with her skin microbiome. And then there's breastmilk, which for many decades was also considered sterile, but which is in fact a creamy bacterial soup (par. 9).

Individuals, thus, acquire a microbiome as an ongoing process of bodily interpenetration amid bodily disambiguation; the process of developing as an autonomously embodied person is also a process of bodily permeability. As babies' introduction to the microbial world, the maternal body serves as a conduit into other forms of environmental relations, and sets the groundwork (perhaps) for future health development. Through translating complex microbiological data into publicly legible media, maternal-fetal microbial attachments are represented as spaces of sociality—the placenta as an introductory venue, the birthing canal as a tourist passage between familiar and strange worlds, and skin-to-skin contact as an embrace.

Noel Mueller and colleagues' 2015 review article in *Trends in Molecular Medicine* titled "The Infant Microbiome Development: Mom Matters" echoes this theme and again relies on a doubled implication of "matter": moms matter as the fleshy material in which fetuses develop and as centrally consequential (molecular) caregivers. Surveying the breadth of emergent research and pointing toward future directions (particularly the possibility of manipulating the microbiome to enhance health outcomes), the authors stress the centrality of "mom." Throughout, the maternal body emerges only through its role as a colonizing force—microbial relations are once again positioned as material and as materializing—and maternal embodiment in effect bears the weight of a child's outcomes. Furthermore, throughout their analysis of how moms matter, the authors shift seamlessly from biological attachments to social nurturance; uterine or vaginal interiority, and breast exteriority are rendered commensurate forms of attachment. Crucially, the scholars do not differentiate between pre- and postnatal relations, as they stress the importance of both vaginal childbirth and breastfeeding on the development of a complex infant microbiome. The linguistic shift from "maternal" (as a form of material relationality) to "mom" (as a form of social relationality) works dynamically to expand how mothers are tasked with responsible embodiment. For although prenatal microbial relations fit neatly into the model of embodied maternal responsibility outlined by Oaks and Armstrong, postnatal relations through breastfeeding and skin contact suggest an elaboration of what formerly counted as maternal embodiment.

In another extension of maternal embodiment, translational medicine researchers are now turning toward ways to make moms' matter itself. Connecting innovative lab research to extant anxieties about the biomedicalization of birth and global epidemiological trends toward increasing rates of Caesarean births, Maria Dominquez-Bello's work on clinical applications of research about the importance of vaginal seeding extends the maternal microbiome extra-corporeally ("Partial Restoration of the Microbiota"). This research draws on hypotheses that the vaginal microbiome is important to answering epidemiological questions about the association between Caesarean births and higher odds of asthma, allergies, and other metabolic conditions (Mueller et al.). In clinical trials before a planned Caesarean birth, researchers inserted sterile gauze into the woman's vagina for about an hour, and then swabbed the newborn with it within minutes of birth. Tested after a month, these infants' microbiomes were more like those of children delivered vaginally than others delivered surgically (Dominguez-Bello et al., "Partial Restoration of the Microbiota"). Although Dominguez-Bello and her team are careful about the circumspectness of these results,[2] these caveats were by and large left out of popular media coverage—best illustrated by the *Science* headline "How to Give a C-section Baby the Potential Benefits of Vaginal Birth" (Couzin-Frankel). Even as some health professionals continue to debate the efficacy and safety of seeding (Cunnington et al.) and the degree to which birth mode, rather than "exposures and events throughout pregnancy" affects infant microbiome development (Aagaard et al., "Una Destinatio, Viae Diversae"), the idea of vaginal swabbing has been incorporated into discourses of evidence-based parenting. Echoing Lupton's argument that modern parenting culture increasingly tasks pregnant individuals with sorting out public health warnings to mitigate risk and enhance outcomes, accounting for the delivery of one's vaginal microbiome is easily taken up into existing narratives about maternal material relations.

This model reinforces Lappé's argument that postgenomic life sciences address the maternal body as an environment for fetal development and as an ecosystem that is itself shaped in context. It elaborates on the classic "soil" metaphor by positioning the maternal body not as inert and bounded by gestation, but as an alive environmental terrain, which moulds further infant health and development. Academic and public writing about maternal-fetal microbial relations are flush with tropes of colonization and ecosystem restoration extending this metaphor in new directions, just as Collins drew on tropes of "15th century explorers" to demonstrate the import of mapping new landscapes. The infant body is one whose initial colonization by maternal microbes establishes the conditions for all future relations with the world—implicitly reproducing narratives that framed European colonialism as contributing to a more moral and hygienic world (Bashford). Bearing the weight of infant-child outcomes, the maternal microbiome is tasked with a kind of embodied responsibility. Improper colonization (such as due to antibiotic exposure) requires the restorative cultivation of an infant's bodily ecosystems, ideally through breastfeeding. "Mom matters," thus, ultimately retreads longstanding public health campaigns stressing the importance of particular kinds of parenting practices—particularly vaginal birth and breastfeeding—now couched as mattering in terms of emergent science. What public narratives about this research reinforce are pernicious cultural ideas about pregnant women as environments tasked with the social responsibility to optimize their bodies in the service of their fetus-child's best interests.

MicroBirth

If "mom matters" for individual health outcomes, then "moms matter" for population-level ones. And if individually ecosystemic body-persons reflect and reproduce environmental contexts, what are the broader social implications of understanding individual women's bodies within a maternal body politics? Linking microbiome research in academic journals and popular science writing to epidemiological, population-level questions about the rise of "conditions of modernity," the 2014 documentary *Microbirth* (directed by Toni Harman and Alex Wakeford) translates circumspect and descriptive research into consequential claims. Winner of the Grand Prix award at the 2014 Life Sciences Film Festival, the documentary presents global humanity as uniquely imperilled at the apotheosis of human achievement, as the narrator queries over an opening montage, "why is it that at this moment in time, our species has never been sicker?" The answer is internal and external, as the film indicts both individual bodily microbiomes as well as social and industrial antibiotic contexts.

The film draws heavily on interviews with expert researchers to frame a narrative of both existential danger and possible salvation. The former is exemplified by an interview with Martin Blaser (director of the Human Microbiome Project at New York University and professor of translational medicine) as he explains that the world has become a fertile environment for "a rising epidemic of plagues from asthma, to obesity, to allergic diseases ... over the last decades and there's no real sign that it's letting up." Within global health research, these plagues of "noncommunicable diseases" (to which some immunologists add mental health conditions) represent the threat of a particular kind of modernity. In the words of Rodney Dietert (professor of immunotoxicology, Cornell University), they are part of an unsustainable project of "creating an invalid society." Stretching from descriptors of individual bodily health, the film draws on predictions from the World Economic Forum and Harvard School of Public Health that these "modernity plagues" have the potential to "bankrupt" global health organizations by 2030, when they will have an estimate global cost of 47 trillion dollars. Thus, individual bodily status is first framed as socially—and economically—consequential, and then molecularly materialized as illustrative of dangerous human practices.

Explaining the nature of becoming human as a process of coevolution with our symbiotic microbes, the film ties a global gut microbiome to the onset of metabolic transitions in the twentieth century and to shifts in industrial, urban, and medical life—what Blaser has coined the "disappearing microbiota hypothesis." Not only has a rapid rise in antibiotic and antibacterial overuse changed our collective microbiomes, but now research demonstrates the intergenerational implications of such shifts. Once again, microbiome research demonstrates the inextricability of human body-persons *in* ecosystemic context and human body-persons *as* ecosystemic context. Furthermore, individual microbial contexts are now framed as having a global social and economic impact.

Turning back to the micro relations of microbiota, the film reiterates that the acquisition of the mother's bacteria is the "first introduction to the world of microbiota, the world we live in" over footage of home birthing scenes. Here this new microbiological research meets the ongoing medical, social, and activist "natural vs. surgical" birth debates. Breastfeeding, the next stage of material relation, is framed as a moment that "sets the template for future life" (Lesley Page, professor of midwifery). Maternal bodies now mediate the question of whether this child "experiences a life filled with health, or one filled with disease" (Dietert). In this presentation the maternal microbiome is no longer an environment that *contributes* to fetal-infant development, but one that *determines* life course outcomes. Although "tomorrow's generation may be on the edge of a precipice," the film says, scientists' microscopic observations of other harmonious ecosystems provide the tools to understand these health threats as filtered through our own selves as "walking ecosystems." As individual people, our bodies carry the weight of inherited social and environmental histories, and as bounded microbiomes, women's bodies are tasked with passing on good histories to the next generation. Though neutral and descriptive in the lab and contextualized within extant narratives about the centrality of maternal responsibility, such formulation boxes women into a paradoxical relationship with their maternal microbiomes.

The point of this analysis is not to question the importance, sincerity, or validity of such research, but rather to emphasize that narratives about maternal embodiment are themselves consequential. The scientists of *Microbirth* repeat that the best gift a mother can give her new baby is "the set up for a healthy future"—a future mediated quite literally by her body. This vision of maternal embodiment reproduces familiar discourses holding women intimately responsible for their children's health and safety, and the fraught political and symbolic terrain of birth-method-choice in which "natural" and "surgical" are given individual and social moral import. The repetition of "natural" to characterize mothering practices, such as breastfeeding and vaginal delivery, obscures the often fraught and personal circumstances in which decisions about them take place. Constructed as a "gift," exposure to a so-called good maternal microbiome becomes a kind of voluntary and volitional offering, one whose quality is under one's control. This suggests that although individual women's bodies may reflect broader social contexts, they as individuals (rather than problematic social contexts) are ultimately responsible for intergenerational microbial inheritance, and, therefore, child life-course outcomes.

When connected to the film's initial questions about species survival and the social-economic costs of population health, formerly descriptive and circumspect research presents maternal bodies as responsive to individual contexts yet responsible for some larger collective. This is perhaps best exemplified a narrator query mid-film:

> But what happens if one generation gives birth by Caesarean section? This could be breaking the chain of maternal connection. Could we be producing a generation of children who are missing bacteria? And could that be passed down and down for all future generations? What is not known is what the consequences of this could be for humanity.

Couched in subjunctive possibility, *Microbirth* frames the need for further population-level research on the long-term outcomes of medical interventions around birth in maternal embodiment that bears the weight of the global world. It is telling that the film ends by making this link explicit. The narrator points out that amid growing acknowledgment by global institutions of the threat noncommunicable diseases pose to national security, there is little acknowledgment of the link between birth method and immune-related conditions. Rendering macro- and micro-ecosystems analogous, filmmakers present both as under threat because of human (in)action by pairing images of severe climate destruction with interviews about internal climate devastation. As the narrator concludes, "let's not make the same mistakes again, let's not wait decades before taking action ... before the global community wakes up to what we may be doing to ourselves, and it all starts with birth." As the film illustrates, this promising life sciences and epidemiological research has material and global implications, and deserves greater public attention and funding. However, its reliance on the subjunctive conjectural—the "could" that extends individual life course to global health security—reproduces narratives positioning maternal embodiment as a bounded environment that contextualizes fetal-child outcomes, but is not itself contextualized within larger social, political, and economic contexts.

This parallels Richardson's conclusion about epigenetics: "it brings the 'environment'—transduced through the maternal body—into processes of biomedicalization, optimization, and manipulation of life initiated by the twentieth-century molecular life sciences" (227). As women's bodies are rendered in environments for fetal-child outcomes, there is no concurrent attention to the ways poverty, racial discrimination, or social stratification may influence women's own environments. The absence of a broader structural frame reproduces a neoliberal model of motherhood (Lupton) in which individual women bear the weight of making responsible choices in the service of a social good. This focus on individual responsibility at first seems ironic given postgenomic life sciences' emphasis on human and non-human relations in context, yet it speaks to the traction of particular models of embodied motherhood as central metaphors in science writing.

Bearing the Weight of the World

Although microbiome researchers are proposing new and exciting models of the body-person as relational and dynamic environments, they do not do so in a cultural vacuum. As popular science writing about human microbiome discourse casts women as environments, it draws on longstanding and politicized cultural narratives about how to understand motherhood and how to regulate maternal health, birth, and childrearing as mothering practices. Rather than particular to this particular branch of the life sciences, this analysis suggests the broad traction of "sleeping metaphors in science" (Martin, "Romance of the Egg and Sperm") is connected to cultural discourses about the "naturalness" of maternal responsibility and caregiving. As Richardson concludes about epigenetics' reliance on such metaphors, "it *resonates* with the history of highly politicized conceptions of maternal responsibility and may further extend biomedical manipulation and social control of the reproductive female body" (my emphasis, 228). Even as emergent research offers new models of how to understand our embodied selves as in relation, some kinds of relations resonate as obviously materially consequential.

These discourses are not neutral. As research points to the influence of the maternal vaginal microbiome on seeding babies' gut colonies and future health, maternal embodiment is once again simultaneously site of connection, potential, and harm. It is not surprising that Dominguez-Bello's initial clinical trial—one she emphasized was preliminary—quickly made the front page of the science section of every major news source because it fit within a larger set of discourses (and argument) about birth method as a kind of responsible motherhood practice. A month later, an article's characterization of vaginal swabbing as a "trend" (Hill) perhaps best illustrates its escalation from academic analysis to public consciousness. Anecdotally, I found myself drawing on my research into the controversies over study design and the circumspectness of the original research claims to console a friend when she found out that she needed a course of antibiotics during labour and worried that her child would lack a so-called good vaginal seeding. Giving children a strong microbial introduction to the world has clearly entered the public consciousness of a particular kind of evidence-based pregnancy advice. If pregnancy is felt in and through the body, then part of the subjective experience is learning to tie maternal microbiotic embodiment to mothering practices.

None of this is problematic on its surface. But as the "mattering" of maternal embodiment shifts from the personal relations of vaginal birth and breastfeeding to the population-level relations in moral panics about metabolic condition, the maternal microbiome is tasked with our intimate and collective future. Thus, it is important to pull out the implicit cultural politics of such research as it is placed in the context of broader discourses about women and their bodies—as gendered embodiment is framed as always already potentially maternal (Waggoner) and as maternal embodiment is always already potentially harmful (Lupton). Though not explicitly connected to maternal relations, when an editorial headline can plausibly state "The Entire Indian Subcontinent Needs a Stool Transplant" (Juthani-Mehta), it is clear that individual women's microbiomes are implicated in the politics of the body politic. When conditions of modernity are framed as problems "seeded by" women's bodily environments, narratives about microbiome research seed a future that itself reproduces pernicious ideas about maternal responsibility as (literally) bearing the weight of the world.

Endnotes

1 This statistic has now been challenged on the basis of reanalysis of the proportion of red blood cells to fecal material; however, it remains one of the key public narratives about the materiality of the microbiota human.

2 The initial study involved seven children delivered vaginally and eleven children delivered surgically, four of whom received the intervention.

Works Cited

Aagaard, Kjersti, et al. "A Metagenomic Approach to Characterization of the Vaginal Microbiome Signature in Pregnancy." *PloS ONE*, vol. 7, no. 6, 2012, pp. 1-15.

Aagaard, Kjersti, et al. "The Placenta Harbors a Unique Microbiome." *Science Translational Medicine*, vol. 6, no. 237, 2014, pp. 237ra65.

Aagaard, Kjersti, et al. "Una Destinatio, Viae Diversae: Does Exposure to the Vaginal Microbiota Confer Health Benefits to the Infant, and Does Lack of Exposure Confer Disease Risk?" *EMBO Reports*, vol. 17, no. 12, 2016, pp. 1679-84.

Allsworth, Jenifer E, et al. "Viral Sexually Transmitted Infections and Bacterial Vaginosis: 2001-2004 National Health and Nutrition Examination Survey Data." *Sexually Transmitted Diseases*, vol. 35, no. 9, 2008, pp. 791-96.

Almeling, Rene, and Miranda R Waggoner. "More and Less than Equal: How Men Factor in the Reproductive Equation." *Gender & Society*, vol. 27, no. 6, 2013, pp. 821-42.

Armstrong, Elizabeth M. *Conceiving Risk, Bearing Responsibility: Fetal Alcohol Syndrome and the Diagnosis of Moral Disorder*. Johns Hopkins University Press, 2003.

Bäckhed, Roswall, et al. "Dynamics and Stabilization of the Human Gut Microbiome during the First Year of Life." *Cell Host and Microbe*, vol. 17, no. 5, 2015, pp. 690-703.

Bashford, Alison. "Global Biopolitics and the History of World Health." *History of the Human Sciences*, vol. 19, no. 1, 2006, pp. 67-88.

Beckett, Katherine. "Fetal Rights and 'Crack Moms': Pregnant Women in the War on Drugs." *Contemporary Drug Problems*, vol. 22, no. 4, 1995, pp. 587-612.

Benezra, Amber. "Datafying Microbes: Malnutrition at the Intersection of Genomics and Global Health." *BioSocieties*, vol. 11, no. 3, 2016, pp. 334-51.

Benezra, Amber, et al. "Anthropology of Microbes." *Proceedings of the National Academy of Sciences*, vol. 109, no. 17, 2012, pp. 6378-81.

Casper, Monica J. *The Making of the Unborn Patient: A Social Anatomy of Fetal Surgery*. Rutgers University Press, 1998.

Couzin-Frankel, Jennifer. "How to Give a C-Section Baby the Potential Benefits of Vaginal Birth." *Science Magazine*, 2016, www.

sciencemag.org/news/2016/02/how-give-c-section-baby-potential-benefits-vaginal-birth. Accessed 19 July 2018.

Cunnington, Aubrey J, et al. "'Vaginal Seeding' of Infants Born by Caesarean Section." *BMJ: British Medical Journal*, vol. 352, 2016, pp. i227.

Delaney, Carol. "The Meaning of Paternity and the Virgin Birth Debate." *Man*, vol. 21, no. 3, 1986, 494-513.

Daniels, Cynthia R. "Between Fathers and Fetuses: The Social Construction of Male Reproduction and the Politics of Fetal Harm." *Signs: Journal of Women in Culture and Society*, vol. 22, no. 3, 1997, pp. 579-616.

Dominguez-Bello, Maria G, et al. "Delivery Mode shapes the Acquisition and Structure of the Initial Microbiota Across Multiple Body Habitats in Newborns." *Proceedings of the National Academy of Sciences*, vol. 107, no. 26, 2010, pp. 11971-75.

Dominguez-Bello, Maria G, et al. "Partial Restoration of the Microbiota of Cesarean-Born Infants via Vaginal Microbial Transfer." *Nature Medicine*, vol. 22, no. 3, 2016, 250-53.

Grens, Kerry. "The Maternal Microbiome: Moms Bombard Their Babies with Bugs both Before and After They're Born." *The Scientist*, 2014, www.the-scientist.com/daily-news/the-maternal-microbiome-37461. Accessed 19 July 2018.

Hill, Milli. "Vaginal 'Seeding': Could this New Birth Trend Be Putting Babies at Risk?" *The Telegraph*, 2016, www.telegraph.co.uk/health-fitness/body/vaginal-seeding-could-this-new-birth-trend-be-putting-babies-at/. Accessed 19 July 2018.

Hickey, Roxana J, et al. "Understanding Vaginal Microbiome Complexity from an Ecological Perspective." *Translational Research*, vol. 160, no. 4, 2012, pp. 267-82.

Juthani-Mehta, Manisha. The Entire Indian Subcontinent Needs a Stool Transplant. *Pacific Standard*, 2015. psmag.com/health-and-behavior/the-entire-indian-subcontinent-needs-a-stool-transplant. Accessed 19 July 2018.

Lappé, Martine, and Hannah Landecker. "How the Genome got a Life Span." *New Genetics and Society*, vol. 34, no. 2, 2015, pp. 152-76.

Lappé, Martine. "The Maternal Body as Environment in Autism Science." *Social Studies of Science*, vol. 46, no. 5, 2016, pp. 675-700.

Lupton, Deborah. "'Precious Cargo': Foetal Subjects, Risk and

Reproductive Citizenship." *Critical Public Health*, vol. 22, no. 3, 2012, pp. 329-40.

Mackendrick, Norah. "More Work for Mother: Chemical Body Burdens as a Maternal Responsibility." *Gender & Society*, vol. 28, no. 5, 2014, 705-28.

Maher, JaneMaree, et al. "Framing the Mother: Childhood Obesity, Maternal Responsibility and Care." *Journal of Gender Studies*, vol. 19, no. 3, 2010, pp. 233-47.

Mauss, Marcel. "A Category of the Human Mind: the Notion of the Person; the Notion of the Self." *The Category of the Person: Anthropology, Philosophy, History*, edited by Stephen Lukes, Cambridge University Press, 1985, pp. 1-25.

Martin, Emily. "The Egg and the Sperm: How Science has constructed a Romance based on Stereotypical Male-Female Roles." *Signs: Journal of Women in Culture and Society*, vol.16, no. 3, 1991, pp. 485-501.

Martin, Emily. *The Woman in the Body: A Cultural Analysis of Reproduction*. Beacon Press, 1997.

McNaughton, Darlene. "From the Womb to the Tomb: Obesity and Maternal Responsibility." *Critical Public Health*, vol. 21, no. 2, 2011, pp. 179-90.

Microbirth. Directed by Toni Harman and Alex Wakeford, Alto Films, 2014.

Mueller, Noel T, et al. "The Infant Microbiome Development: Mom Matters." *Trends in Molecular Medicine*, vol. 21, no. 2, 2015, pp. 109-117.

National Institutes of Health (NIH). "NIH Human Microbiome Project Defines Normal Bacterial Makeup of the Body: Genome Sequencing Creates First Reference Data for Microbes Living with Healthy Adults." *National Institute of Health*, 2012, www.nih.gov/news-events/news-releases/nih-human-microbiome-project-defines-normal-bacterial-makeup-body. Accessed 19 July 2018.

Oaks, Laury. "Smoke-Filled Wombs and Fragile Fetuses: The Social Politics of Fetal Representation." *Signs: Journal of Women in Culture and Society*, vol. 26, no. 1, 2000, pp. 63-108.

Pitts-Taylor, Victoria. "Mattering: Feminism, Science, and Corporeal Politics" *Mattering: Feminism, Science, and Materialism*, edited by Victoria Pitts-Taylor, New York University Press, 2016, pp. 1-21.

Powell, Kendall. "The Superhero in the Vagina: Can Researchers Harness the Power of Protective Bacteria to Guard against a Common Infection?" *The Atlantic*, 2016, www.theatlantic.com/health/archive/2016/10/the-superhero-in-the-vagina/503720/. Accessed 19 July 2018.

Richardson, Sarah. "Maternal Bodies in the Postgenomic Order." *Postgenomics Perspective on Biology after the Genome*, edited by Sarah Richardson and Hallam Stevens, Duke University Press, 2015, pp. 210-31.

Segata, Nicola. "Gut Microbiome: Westernization and the Disappearance of Intestinal Diversity." *Current Biology*, vol. 25, no. 14, 2015, pp. R611-R613.

Stewart, Christopher J, et al. "Cesarean or Vaginal Birth Does Not Impact the Longitudinal Development of the Gut Microbiome in a Cohort of Exclusively Preterm Infants." *Frontiers in Microbiology*, vol. 8, 2017, pp. 1008-16.

Weir, Lorna. *Pregnancy, Risk and Biopolitics: On the Threshold of the Living Subject*. Routledge, 2006.

Waggoner, Miranda R. "Cultivating the Maternal Future: Public Health and the Prepregnant Self." *Signs: Journal of Women in Culture and Society*, vol. 40, no. 4, 2015, pp. 939-62.

Warin, Megan, et al. "Mothers as Smoking Guns: Fetal Overnutrition and the Reproduction of Obesity." *Feminism and Psychology*, vol. 22, no. 3, 2012, pp. 360-75.

Yatsunenko, Tanya, et al. "Human Gut Microbiome Viewed Across Age and Geography." *Nature*, vol. 486, no. 7402, 2012, pp. 222-27.

Yong, Ed. "There Is No 'Healthy' Microbiome." *New York Times*, 2014, www.nytimes.com/2014/11/02/opinion/sunday/there-is-no-healthy-microbiome.html. Accessed 19 July 2018.

Chapter Six

The Temporality of Maternal Embodiment and the Creative Process: Project *Transit Spaces*

Ruchika Wason Singh

Transit Spaces is a body of work I created through my 2002 pregnancy and thereafter. It consists of paintings reflecting my joy of maternal embodiment, an experience that was both biological and emotional. The project weaves the lived experience of body as a space of transit (for my yet-to-be-born child). It deals with the body as a site for a temporal experience of material embodiment, which is recreated as an artistic expression in this project.

The works in the project are intuitive in nature. I did not follow a structure or create any planned stages for myself; there are no direct correspondences to the stages of pregnancy. Rather, it was the gradual progression of my pregnancy and its experience, alongside which my forms evolved. For a period of nine months, my body spontaneously performed two creative processes: the internal creation of my daughter Meher and the external making of my art. Each operated parallel to the other; each complemented and positively affected the other.

With the shifts in my biological state, I desired to express and emote the joyful knowledge of maternal embodiment. The nature of the works was also affected by activities I engaged in during pregnancy. I began looking at images from the field of microbiology. Browsing through them without understanding their deep scientific meaning, I developed a connection with them. I also found myself engaging in gardening and plantation. Both of these activities had affiliations with the processes of germination, growth, as well as with nurturing and caretaking—my ongoing states.

Subconsciously, I realized that my artistic expression was shaped by my not knowing about the gender of my yet to be born child. In *Transit Spaces*, I made this ambiguity instead a thing of beauty by using metaphor as a key visual tool. Amoebic forms and botanical formations helped me maintain the pleasant tension of wanting to express what was not yet known to me. Initially, I played with them as singular and smaller forms. I drew with graphite on paper. Gradually, the expression evolved into a painterly articulation, in which the doodles and sketches expressed the experience of maternal embodiment beyond a quick visual note, a scribble, or a sketch. I worked with acrylic paint on *shikishi* (traditional Japanese paper called *washi* pasted on a board) and canvas. Although I introduced colour into my imagination of maternal embodiment, my work mainly remained monochromatic. Colour played a conceptual role here, as my choice of crimson and reds was synonymous with blood and flesh. With such a colour selection, I created what I would like to call an "altered botany of maternal embodiment," which powerfully opposes a teleologically constructed imagination.

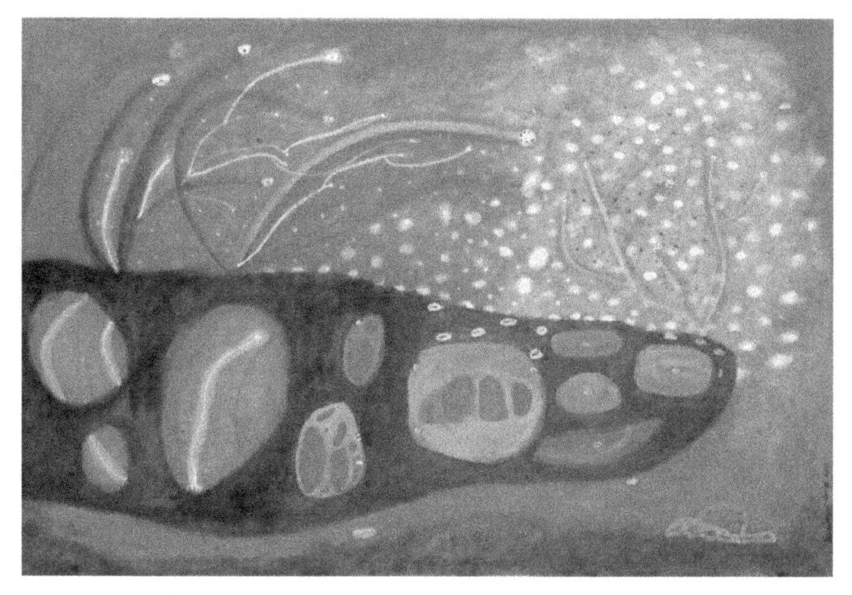

Figure 1. Transit Spaces image. Being and Becoming I • Acrylic on Shikishi • 38.1cm x 57.15cm, 2004

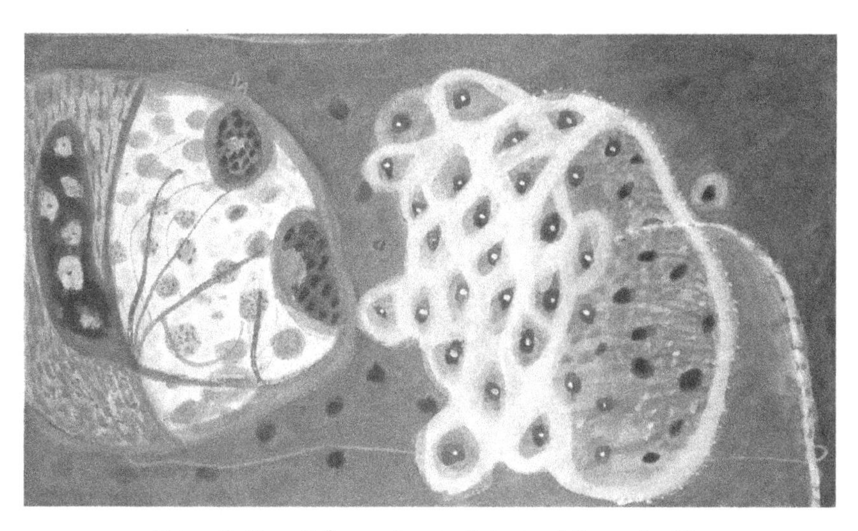

Figure 2. Transit Spaces image. Being and Becoming II • • Acrylic on Shikishi • 22cm x 38.1cm, 2004

Chapter Seven

Embodied Governance: Community Health, Indigenous Self-Determination, and Birth Practices

Erynne M. Gilpin and Sarah Marie Wiebe

Authors' Self-Location

Erynne M. Gilpin: *As an Indigenous researcher, community member, and birth worker (doula) of mixed ancestry (Saulteaux-Cree Métis (Treaty 5), Filipina, Irish, and Scottish), I am who I am related to and, furthermore, to the Land and Water that raised me and my people. This reflection, among others, represents ongoing reflections and conversations with family and extended community. For myself, my academic, creative, and activist work extend out of my own expanding consciousness and personal commitments toward decolonial ways of being and becoming. In writing this piece, I acknowledge the unceded Coast Salish and Straits territories and waters on which I work and learn as uninvited guest. Nitatαminan for the kindness, mentorship, and guidance from all teachers, supervisors, and old ones in my life. I raise my hands to the knowledge keepers, Land and Water defenders, and birth workers of these territories and give thanks for the opportunity to exist and grow in your ancestral landscapes.*

Sarah Marie Wiebe: *Across the Pacific Ocean, this academic journey has taken me from unceded Coast Salish and Straights territories to Honolulu, Hawai'i, where I have the privilege of teaching, researching, and collaborating with brilliant minds to challenge settler-colonialism and envision decolonial futures. As a non-Indigenous Canadian raised on unceded Tsleil-Waututh territory along the "Indian Arm" of the Salish Sea, I acknowledge the responsibilities I carry to the peoples and places informing the person I am today. In my view, writing is one form of academic-activism that aims to unsettle ongoing colonial processes. Working together in pursuit of an ongoing process of decolonization, it is an honour to share this process of writing with Erynne and to be in conversation with each other about how bodies are vital sites of resurgence and regeneration. I am grateful to the Centre for Global Studies at the University of Victoria for creating space for these conversations and appreciate the opportunities Erynne and I have had to visit with communities and to learn about reproductive justice, embodied governance, and cultural renewal.*

> "While community wellness and healing are intricately tied to contemporary demands for self-government, there is very little written that addresses the relationship between self-determination and communities in crisis."—Ladner 88

Despite the prevalence of widespread narratives positioning Indigenous health and bodies as in crisis, Indigenous peoples across Turtle Island and around the world are reclaiming health and wellness practices. This reclamation, we suggest, reveals a radical form of cultural resurgence and self-determination. In this paper, we argue for a framework of "embodied governance," which brings together Indigenous wellness, governance, and gender analyses to counter the notion of the Indigenous body as in need of a health intervention. We understand embodied governance as a renewed understanding of governance—one that centres the rebirth of community culture, ceremony, and protocol, resists extraction, and emphasizes regeneration, resurgence, restorying, restoration, and renewal. We focus on the body as a crucial site for self-determination. In doing so, we reposition the Indigenous body as a site of cultural renewal and regeneration. Regenerative health requires that Indigenous peoples decide for themselves how to govern their bodies and "promote more life" on their own terms (Simpson 141). In this chapter, as community-engaged academic-activist scholars, we discuss the importance of participating in healing research methodologies and practices that "explicitly engage and enact the cultural knowledge, historical and traditional wisdom, politics and ever-present spiritualities" (Chilisa 278). We take seriously the importance of reproductive bodies— including a range of embodied, experiential, place-based, and caretaking roles across genders— within a framework bringing together critical Indigenous studies, Indigenous governance, and reproductive justice. These ideals are not constricted to gendered notions of femaleness; rather, they require a personal commitment for all community members to protect and pass on cultural teachings to future generations. The discussion of embodied governance presented here intends to interrogate colonial reproductions of sexualized violence, which imposes gender binaries, heteronormativity, and frameworks of patriarchy. It also works to centre Indigenous conceptions of gender fluidity, embodied relational experience, and self-determined sexualities through relational practices grounded in culture, kinship, and care.

This chapter identifies four central pillars assisting in ongoing discussions and investigations of Indigenous governance traditions: accountability, relationship, cultural safety, and women's leadership. These concepts provide a framework from which we can engage in ongoing efforts of personal, community, Land/Water-based healing for the purpose of protecting the future for generations to come. Our analysis contributes to this discussion by celebrating and honouring on-the-ground practices of self-determination, and by focusing on rooted examples of community birth work, which builds upon Erynne's doctoral research.

The wellness of Indigenous people is dependent upon the wellness of the environment, including territories encompassing Land[1] and Water. Land provides us with an ontological framework for understanding relationships and relational accountability. Land and Water teach us about our interdependent states of being, in relation to one another, and, furthermore, provide us with the protocols to uphold and respect these relationships. Glen Coulthard reminds us that the "the Land occupies an ontological framework for understanding relationships" (1)—including the enactment of relationship to self, others, spirit, and the Land/Waters—and ultimately constitutes Indigenous conception of good governance and health. Certainly, as the recent health concerns in Attawapiskat highlighted, when eleven youth attempted to take their own lives, there are widespread and diverse crises among Indigenous communities, which are the direct result of systemic violence. Yet as we have discussed in the Reimagining Attawapiskat project (see www.reimaginingattawapiskat.com), these are not the only stories about Indigenous communities. Although we orient our attention to possibilities for brighter and decolonial futures, we are mindful of the ongoing legacy of colonialism and gendered realities affecting overall community wellness. These include the violent loss of so many women and girls, suicide epidemics among youth, intergenerational trauma from residential schools, inexcusable lack of access to clean Water, and so many other untold stories of loss, disconnection, and hopelessness (Halseth; Ladner; NWAC; Stout). As further outlined in the 1996 Royal Commission on Aboriginal Peoples (RCAP) final report, Indigenous women "have often been excluded from their home communities, from decision-making, and from having a say in their future and their children's future.... As Aboriginal people develop and implement self-government, the perspectives of Aboriginal women must guide them" (95-96). All are explicit indicators of the pervasiveness of colonialism today and the ongoing sexualized violence enacted on the bodies and hearts of Indigenous women, girls, two-spirit community members, and trans folk. In her work *Therapeutic Nations: Healing in an Age of Indigenous Rights*, Tanana Athabascan scholar Diane Million discerns that "gender inequality and gender violence haunt the constitution of new polities in the articulation of any Indigenous self-determination"; thus, we have to understand "the increasing gender violence perpetrated against Indigenous women as more than an attack on individuals, and as a mobile but durable feature of colonial power relations" (7). These processes not only affect community health and wellness, they simultaneously undermine traditional governance systems. In this respect, the loss of Land and identity ultimately affects Indigenous health. Women are uniquely situated in these processes of cultural dislocation. By discussing this contextual history and by then centring embodied governance, we emphasize both heartbreak and hope in the unfinished, ongoing, and unsettled process of decolonization.

There are systemic barriers to the meaningful political participation of Indigenous women in systems of governance, which have consequences for community health and self-determination. In general, there exists a lack of understanding about what we can learn from Indigenous women's insights about the transformation of governance and healing models. This rupture is in part due to the effects of colonialism on the lives of Indigenous women today, which translate into higher rates of physical gendered and sexualized violence on the female body. Indigenous women are five times more likely to die as result of violence than non-Indigenous women, and three times more likely to commit suicide than Canadian women (Halseth; Ladner; NWAC; Stout). Colonial gendered violence, whether in the form of a perpetrator or through manifested hopelessness, actively tears through the homes and hearts of Indigenous families. Even though missing and murdered women, as well as their affected families and impacted communities, bear the scars of marginalization, violence, and systemic apathy, Indigenous women continue to demonstrate strength and renewal in ways countering colonial damage (Hunt; Jiménez-Altamirano-Jiménez; RCAP section 3; Simpson). They will not be silenced.

Indigenous women bear intimate relationships to the Land and Water, which position them as optimal leaders for Land- and Water-based healing and authentic community governance. It is through their connections with Land that Indigenous women source their strength to lead, protect, teach, birth, and love their communities. A woman's intimate connection to the Land and Water also makes her vulnerable to the aggressive extraction of natural resources and facilitated Land theft for the purpose of neoliberal capitalist expansion. As the Native Youth Sexual Health Network (NYSHN) poignantly emphasizes, the extractive industry in Canada, ranging from pipeline construction to mining projects, happens within a social context affecting the everyday lives of many who live with the consequences of these industrial developments. A gendered lens inspired by the insights offered by NYSHN reveals how those at the frontlines experience the intergenerational effects because of multiple projects affecting Lands, Waters, and bodies. Women and children living at the frontlines of these developments often experience the devastating impacts of environmental contamination firsthand, which range from contaminated breastmilk to elevated levels of contaminants and reproductive cancers. In this respect, the ill health of the environment has significant consequences for the health of communities and their ability to pass on cultural knowledge to future generations.

Although existing research continues to explore the links between governance and health, the leadership potential of women is not fully acknowledged, even though Indigenous governance traditions are predicated on women's central role. An embodied governance framework begins with a celebration of women and their contributions to self-determining governing systems. We also acknowledge the importance of intersectional analysis and centring community within this framework. As Sandy Grande (Quechua) proclaims, defense of Land translates into defense of Indigenous women and knowledge because "we can not have strong nations without strong women" (gtd. in Alfred 95). It is necessary to be more explicit above what many of the authors, activists, and researchers have emphasized as integral qualities of Indigenous governance and wellness leadership. Million states that Indigenous women are "creating new language for communities to address the real multilayered facets of their histories and concerns by insisting on the inclusion of [their] lived experience, rich with emotional knowledges, of what pain and grief and hope meant or mean now in our pasts and futures" (57); this is what Million refers to as felt theory: "felt experience as community knowledge; knowledge is "affective, felt, intuited as well as thought" (57). Honouring this felt knowledge while situated across the Pacific Ocean between Hawai'i and Coast Salish territories of the Wasanec, Sonhgees, and Esquimalt Nations, we raise our hands to local efforts of women-led Land-centred community wellbeing initiatives—such as the Tsartlip First Nation Community Garden Project, Land revitalization efforts of Tsartlip First Nation's Project Reclaim, and the Ekw'í7tl Indigenous Doula Collective. These initiatives, among others, demonstrate that Land- and Water-based cultural protocols and women-centred leadership enact living networks of personal and collective governance, which moves through the very bodies of those on the Land.

To build a framework of embodied (felt, lived, and experienced) governance—which is grounded in community and centred upon renewal and regeneration, and resists an extractive approach to resources such as Land and Water—this chapter first explains the extractivist settler-colonial context and mentality or colonial governmentality (Coulthard), which have enabled some of the ongoing injustices experienced by Indigenous bodies today. We begin with an interrogation of colonial forces proliferating in the context of healthcare with the aim of disrupting health inequities faced by Indigenous peoples. Anchored in an analysis of birth-work practice and women's leadership, our intervention into the colonial healthcare field tries to recentre the Indigenous body as a radical site of regeneration, knowledge, and governance.

Beyond Colonial Governmentality

Many illnesses within Indigenous communities arise from social, economic, and political inequalities, stemming from a history of colonialism (Chad et al.; Mundel and Chapman). Colonization is the root cause of the loss of linguistic, cultural, and identity strength, all of which establish the foundation of traditional political governance models and practice (Alfred; Corntassel 2; Kirmayer et al.; Simpson). Frantz Fanon has articulated that colonialism is an internalized process, which normalizes conditioned ways of understanding ethico-political norms and practice... When interpreted through a framework of physical infestation, colonial imperialism transcends the domain of theoretical abstraction and becomes more pragmatically understood at the level of everyday action and felt through the body.

We can understand the intimate effects of this colonial formulation through the following processes. Land and Water inform Indigenous ontologies, relationships, and healing. Colonial expansion and capitalist extraction are dependent on the perpetual acquisition of Land and cognitive imperialism in order to facilitate Land theft (Altamirano-Jiménez; Coulthard; Simpson). Separation from the Land causes a severing of relationship to culture, language, and ancestral knowledge, which leads to physical and mental illness. This is particularly true for Indigenous communities and Nations who "understand their knowledge as inextricable from their lived experience in their distinct places, in spiritual relationships with land and life, and from traditions that change but are millennial" (Million 13). However, these are not linear relationships or discrete issues, as they are often addressed as such in research. Instead, these elements of governance and healing are recursive, cyclical, and regenerative. Each informs the other. For example, Canada's RCAP defines healing as "personal and societal recovery from the lasting effects of oppression and systemic racism experienced over generations." It continues: "Many Aboriginal people are suffering, not simply from specific diseases and social problems, but also from depression of spirit, resulting from more than 200 years of dismantling of their cultures, language, identities and self-respect" (474). The ability to self-govern and uphold regenerative wellness within Indigenous communities is dependent upon a meaningful relationship to the Land and Water, which needs to be examined and explored in its relational form.

Indigenous governance can be understood as the simultaneous interrogation of contemporary colonialism(s), along with a resurgence of traditional economic, social, political, and spiritual governance systems, which reflects the values and language of a subjective community. The interlocking features of colonial power establish a hierarchy of dominance within Western social, economic, and political institutions. These systems condition what Charlotte Loppie defines as proximal (interpersonal, direct relationship), intermediate (social, community), and distal (systemic, societal, historical, and/or institutional) determinants of health. As she further explains: "the circumstances in which people are born, grow live work and age are responsible for most of the health inequities that have persisted and widened within and between countries" (4). Because colonial logic is predicated on white supremacist and patriarchal conduct, those regarded as inferior—whether by their race, gender or class—experience vast inequality in their social, political, and economic standing (Halseth), which means the ability to live out their physical, mental, and spiritual wellness is reflective of and impacted by political process. Seminal works—such as Michael J. Chandler and Christopher Lalonde's findings that community health (with a focus on suicide prevention) was a function of their degree of autonomy and self-government, Laurence J. Kirmayer's contributions toward Land-based healing methodologies, or Taiaiake Alfred's proposal for a decolonized framework for self-betterment based on "one warrior at a time"—contribute to efforts that locate Indigenous healing traditions at the heart of Indigenous governance methodologies and praxis. In this way, taking care of our own mental, physical, spiritual, and emotional Landscapes is deeply embedded in larger relational networks of care and community wellbeing. As Shirley Tagalik asserts, "cultural wellbeing relies on the individual becoming situated within a cultural worldview" (1); in this way, when we care for ourselves, our families, and communities, we care for our Nations. When situating body as a site of determination and, therefore, governance, individuals are given the opportunity to reflect critically about the ways in which they can uphold their own unique responsibilities and gifts within larger collective efforts to generate community wellbeing and governance.

Determining Indigenous Health Futures

There are numerous and multidimensional ways to transmit knowledge about health, bodies, and governance. Leanne Simpson (Anishinaabe), among others, notes that the responsibilities of Indigenous scholars should transcend the mere documentation of knowledge and locate their physical bodies on the Land (Alfred; Corntassel 1; Salmón). When we as researchers are situated on our home territories, or in the territories of the communities we serve, or are students of, we have access and therefore responsibilities, to community protocol. Coulthard (Yellowknives Dene) describes how Land occupies an ontological framework for how we engage in relationship with the world around us. He counters colonial and neoliberal assumptions that Land is exclusively a material resource for extraction, and reminds us that it is constitutive to who we are. It is this conception of identity that grounds Indigenous knowledge and relational protocol. Storytelling practices are at the core of Indigenous resurgence efforts to counter extractive colonial governmentalities.

Conceptions of identity, protocol, and relational accountability are passed on through storytelling and storied research methodologies. For Shawn Wilson (Opaskwayak Cree), storied research methodologies provide avenues to "inform our resistance and centre our narrative but also translate information" (98). The stories coming from diverse Landscapes and Seascapes encode the information necessary to enact social protocols, which constitute the integrity of systems of governance. Beyond the colonial imaginary, Indigenous communities and scholars use storytelling methods as avenues of emancipation and liberation, and to tell their own stories on their own terms. Each individual who encounters a story bears witness to it and, thusm is held responsible to interpret the meaning; the story locates the listener in a situation of agency and action. The stories we tell and are told manufacture the imaginatives of political possibility and relational protocol. For Corntassel (1), Chaw-win-is (Nuu-Chah-Nulth), and T'lakwadzi (Kwakwaka'wakw), storytelling is a "starting point for renewing

Indigenous family and community responsibilities in the ongoing struggle for Indigenous justice and freedom" (4), and provides a pathway to imagine beyond colonial relationships and to transform power. Storytelling methodologies allow for individuals to create their own meaning, and when stories are shared and embedded in living histories of a people and place, they provide the space necessary for communities to co-create their ways into a future informed by cultural values and Land- and Water-based knowledges. The languages carrying storied teachings encode the fabric of Indigenous epistemological and ontological unfoldings of relationships and the emergence of political and cultural governance.

The Cree-Michif teachings of Mino-Pimatisiwin are a way to understand "living a good life" or "walking in a good way." They describe how our overall sense of wellbeing is an interconnected process accounting for mental, physical, emotional, and spiritual ways of being. When applied to a political discourse, Indigenous frameworks, such as Mino-Pimatisiwin, find a system of governance premised on balanced relations and relational accountability within all facets of social life. Similarly, we can learn from Nuu-chah-nulth scholar, hereditary Chief, and author Richard Atleo (Nuu-chah-nulth) who shares his own teachings of "*heshook-ish tsawalk*," or "everything is one" in his book *Tsawalk: A Nuu-chah-nulth Worldview*. By positioning himself deeply in his own cultural teachings of Tsawalk, Atleo explores the ways in which Tsawalk provides a framework of relationships between the physical and spiritual. Western systems of health and healing have much to learn from the diverse array of Indigenous approaches to community wellbeing.

Indigenous Governance: Everyday Acts and Beyond

A renewed understanding of governance as an ethic of how we care for ourselves and others enhances our ability to confront ongoing projections of colonialism and position ourselves from a place of mental clarity, physical strength, and emotional courage. Cultural revitalization, political leadership, and community wellbeing within this framework are situated as acts of everyday resurgence: everyday efforts taking place at the kitchen table, on the drive to school, or in the birth room (Corntassel et al.). George Manuel reminds us that "it is necessary to heal ourselves with our own medicine. This is integral in self-determination and insurgent healing" (106). Insurgent healing in this way can be understood as engaging with community healing practices, and as acknowledging that individual healing and self-care requires taking care of oneself in order to best take care of communities and families.

Just as Indigenous research methodologies require a heightened commitment to community accountability, Indigenous healing, and wellness, they also require accountability to the needs, protocols, experiences, and traditional governance of the Indigenous communities involved (Gomes et al.; Kovach; Wilson). Accountability requires intensive and ongoing self-reflection, of the caregiver or community; it prioritizes the needs, language, cultural protocols, and knowledge of the community "if it is to be counted as Indigenous" (Wilson 42). Models of healing and wellness governance must incorporate the wisdom of local elders, heed the voices of ancestral knowledge and be centred around the experience of Indigenous youth (Carson et al.; Gomes et al.; Reimagining Attawapiskat). The translation of cultural knowledge from elders to youth, and from youth to elders, constitutes as a central artery for community cultural strength and embodied governance practices. Intergenerational knowledge requires the full presence of relationship. Knowledge translation requires for the full presence of the mental, physical, spiritual and emotional bodies. cThis knowledge must be grounded in trust, respect, and reciprocity.

Healthy relationships are necessary to actualize authentic models of healing and wellness governance. Linda Smith reminds us that "right relationship and research involves a complex decolonizing process that involved reconciling settler and native relations," including a commitment to anticolonial imperialism as well as transformative relationships between colonizer and the colonized (Gomes et al. 1). This is essential in the delivery of safe, effective, and regenerative wellness and healing practice, as it aims to "cultivate a reciprocal, responsible relationship as a means to making right relationships and providing access to culturally appropriate health systems" (1). Not only must healthcare institutions make space for Indigenous healing knowledge and technologies, but they must mandate space for Indigenous healthcare practitioners and antiracist education for non-Indigenous caregivers.

Cultural relevance is the final pillar of healing traditions as governance we discuss in this chapter. Establishing culture as a central component in the way we engage in healing and wellness practice contributes to enhanced access to health care services and improved outcomes, and honours the dignity and value of Indigenous knowledges and worldviews (Gomes et al.; Halseth). As Carl Hammerschlag states, "healing promotes the idea of bringing together many forces to best utilize the powers that promote health" (qtd. in McCormik 2), and culture is a crucial power toward regenerative wellness and self-determination. The erasure and legalization of Indigenous culture are direct attacks on Indigenous autonomy and nationhood. Recentring culture in our healing traditions can fortify our overall ability to self-govern and exercise meaningful decolonization. Many Indigenous women carry cultural memories and political visions, which constitute the relational backbone of contemporary Indigenous governance. This leads into another central category of Indigenous wellness and healing as governance: women's leadership. Through the lived experiences, voices, and strength of Indigenous women, we can discover meaningful and authentic healing and growth.

Land as Body

For many Indigenous communities, Land is considered as kin, as a relative or relation. Kānaka Maoli scholars describe kin relationships to Land, Water, and place as relationship through "Piko." Piko, like the umbilical cord, connects us to our first home and extends out into relationships, which tie us to Land memories, ancestral Waterways, and place-based knowledge systems of relationship, governance, and ancestral or genealogical belonging (Casumbal-Salazar; Goodyear-Ka'ōpua et al.). Moreover, women embody an intimate relationship to Water and are, therefore, accountable to take care of and uphold relationship to Water. In conversations with elders and communities, Indigenous scholars—such as Kim Anderson, Leanne Simpson, Lee Maracle, and Priscilla Settee—all share stories and reflections centred on the unique relationship and responsibilities that Indigenous women have to and with Water. Women's bodies are intimately interconnected to Water, as it passes through with new life in childbirth, and shares the cycles of the moon with cyclical menstruation cycles (Anderson). In

Cree, the word for Water, "*Nipiy,*" can also mean "life." Cree-Métis elder Tom McCallum explains that to say "death," we actually can say "Nipiyani" or "return to the Water." Water is the life force of all relations, and it is the thread interconnecting our beings, destinies, and futures. Water is the foundation of good health. It possesses healing properties connecting us to constellations of connection with all of Creation. These ideals are not constricted to colonial gendered notions of femaleness or colonial gender binaries; rather, they require a personal commitment for all community members to protect and pass on cultural teachings to future generations. We acknowledge that all bodies embody and reproduce governance practices of resurgence, knowledge translation, relational accountability, and cultural protocol in diverse and meaningful ways.

All people have the ability to reproduce culture for future generations. This connection between physical and cultural reproduction is crucial for the advancement for intergenerational knowledge and reproductive justice (Hoover et al.; NYSHN). In upholding these responsibilities, women have the opportunity to inspire a relational accountability to the Land and Water, and to challenge younger generations to reflect about the ways our ancestors protected the Land and Water.

Vibrant and healthy Indigenous bodies constitute the grounds for thriving and politically autonomous Nations. However, where women centred Indigenous leadership has been recognized, it has been narrowly examined within constricted state-centred notions of political change, negating the yet untapped contributions women-centered Indigenous leadership can give to healing and wellness methods within families, communities, and Nations (Alfred; Kuokkanen; Sunseri; Suzack). There are three indispensable characteristics of Indigenous women's leadership, within the context of healing and wellness, which make the role of women essential to the overall efforts toward political consciousness and liberation: the motherhood paradigm, kincentric models of relations (or *Wahkilhtowin*), and embodied governance (Land as body, Water as blood).

The Motherhood Paradigm

Care and kinship are central to embodied governance. Simpson, among others, discusses the importance of centring motherhood and familial paradigms in their own commitment to personal and collective wellness: "the family is a microcosm of the nation" and how we care for our families determines how we care for our Nation (145). These paradigms establish a framework of relational accountability, which flows from a conscious and intentional relationship to the Land, as Original Mother, and into the politics of motherhood, within the communities themselves. Simpson's notion of breastfeeding as treaty is a landmark contribution to evolving theory of motherhood, parenthood and life-givers as carriers of the Nation. She explains that breastfeeding is a child's first exposure to relationship based on reciprocal exchange, which enables them to learn about "treaties, the relationships they encode and how to maintain good treaty relationships" (108). The fragmentation of family and the undermining of the role of motherhood through colonial political genocide have created a crisis in the need to rebuild strong families.

Cherokee elder Marilou Awaiakta shares that carriers of culture are accountable to the wellbeing and strength of the entire community (Anderson). The ability to regenerate culture is what defines motherhood within this paradigm. The extension of the notion of motherhood and lifegiver has the capacity to complicate and deepen our understanding of kinship and relational accountability. If motherhood is defined by the capacity to carry knowledge for the betterment of the community, our own relationships to Indigenous communities are defined by the responsibilities we possess. This is not unlike Anderson's articulation of Native women as "the embodiment of transformation and change, and when we understand this we can begin to appreciate the responsibility that comes with power" (184).

Wahkihtowin: Kincentric Models of Relationship

Kinship-centred paradigms are what constitute Indigenous political knowledge and healing methodologies. The Cree and Michif teaching of Wahkitowin, or the act of being in kinship or in relationship to one another, provides a framework for being in good relation and for enacting protocols of accountability among all relations (Hancock). It is a practice that acknowledges individual beings are not isolated; they are situated in a constellation of relationality. This conception of relationship extends to the spirit world, to the animal, plant, and medicine Nations, and flows from relationship to Land and Water. We come from the Land, and in turn the Land teaches us the possibilities of how we relate to one another. Relationship as a verb requires consciousness, compassion, and creativity. The political telos of Indigenous consciousness is to restore relationship to self, others, spirit, and the Land through authentic governance and regenerative community health. Recentring women as the embodiment of Land- and Water-based connection forces communities to protect the Land and Water, and to observe a sacred reverence toward the feminine. One way in which Indigenous women across Turtle Island enact a politics of community health wellness is through the active resurgence of traditional birth work, care, and ceremony.

Embodied Governance: Land as Body, Water as Blood

For mothers and families around the world, the ways in which we birth our young babies is an act of sovereignty, self-determination, and ceremony. Here on Turtle Island (Canada), there are strong hands, hearts, and minds dedicating their lives to ensure that Indigenous babies are born in ways upholding their culture, language, ceremony, and the Land. As Canada's 2015 Truth and Reconciliation final report (TRC) emphasized, colonial political genocide has undermined traditional family structures, which displaces women from healing, birthing, and political leadership. The way we govern our bodies in sexuality, traditional food choices, and birthing is an act of self-determination. Indigenous women and birth workers carry cultural memories and political visions, which constitute the relational backbone of contemporary Indigenous governance (Alfred; Kuokkanane; Sunseri; Suzack).

Unfortunately, racism is alive and well within healthcare institutions across Turtle Island (Leyland et al.; Loppie et al.; Kirmayer). It is paramount that Indigenous families and mothers can access care from Indigenous birth workers, midwives, and doulas ("aunties"). As Western medicine, often male dominated, took precedent over Indigenous healing traditions from the mid-1800s to the present day, many traditional healers, often women and two-spirit, were removed from positions of healing authority (Bellrichard; Mundel and Chapman; NAHO). Our teachings, our medicines, our songs, and our ways were regarded as alternative, less scientific, and inadequate for the delivery of healthy and safe births. The ability to self-govern and uphold regenerative wellness within Indigenous communities is dependent upon a meaningful relationship to the Land and Water, which needs to be examined and explored in its relational form. For Indigenous birth workers, relational protocol and teachings surrounding the labour and postpartum chapters of birth are all sites of governance and viable pathways toward shared cultural determination.

The Removal of Birth from Community

For Indigenous families across Turtle Island, it is common for them to leave their home communities about a month before due date and give birth outside their community (Adelson; Health Canada; NWAC; Statistics Canada; Varcoe et al.). There are many challenges preventing Indigenous families from giving birth on their home territories, and although many families feel safer travelling to sites of urbanized healthcare service, giving birth out of community undermines local Indigenous health, birthing, and wellness systems of governance in three ways. First, it prioritizes non-Indigenous healthcare practitioners and practices over local traditions and protocol. Second, the removal of a birth from home territories, Water, elders, and languages affects the ways in which culture can guide birthing ceremonies and governance systems. Birth protocol shifts when families do not have the option of giving birth in their home territories and languages. Finally, when families are not given the option to access safe, culturally led, and Land- and Water-based birth, their own health and governance systems are discredited. The effects of the removal of births from the home territories, Water, and hands of Indigenous communities have had deeply "profound spiritual and cultural consequences, which are difficult to quantify. The loss of traditional birthing practices has been linked to the loss of cultural identity" (NAHO 4).

Birth workers are the keepers of cultural protocols, ancestral knowledge, and Land- and Water-based traditions that situate birthing practice as a model of community, cultural, and body governance. From the Birthing The Nation Project, a culturally grounded prenatal parenting circle at Ho'oulu'āina in Kalihi Valley, Hawaii, to the Seventh Generation Midwives in Toronto, Canada, to the Nesting Doula Collective for Indigenous Families and Families of Colour in territories of the Coast Salish and Lekwungen Speaking Peoples (Victoria B.C.), to the Indigenous Freedom Babies, and to the Indigenous midwives and birth keepers of the "AMUPAKIN Achimamas" in Ecuador—Indigenous birth workers are loving, caring for, protecting, and birthing the Nations around the world. To many Indigenous peoples, the birth of little ones is an act of ceremony. Indigenous birth workers believe that the woman carrying a child is profoundly spiritual and sacred. She is a spiritual entity connecting the elder Kokum-Pîsim to their home Kã wee ooma aski through the rush of nipiy. These teachings remind us that our children are closest to the Spirit World and hold special authority in our communities. As women's bodies are intimately interconnected to Water, it passes through with new life in childbirth, and shares the cycles of the moon with our own cyclical menstruation (Anderson).

As Myrna Laramee highlights, Water "is what connects us" and all beings: "when we are in that circle and that women gets up and passes Water ... she is creating a spiritual umbilical cord, and without her to do that, we just sit as spiritual entities. The minute she passes that Water from soul to soul, you are attached to that central spiritual connection and you can drink from it" (185). For many Indigenous communities, women embody an intimate relationship to Water and are, therefore, accountable to take care of and uphold their relationships to it. Water encodes the instructions we need to care for one another, and give life—whether physically, culturally, socially, and spiritually—to our communities and growing Nations. Indigenous women's intimate relationships to the Land and Water position them as optimal leaders for Land-based healing and authentic community governance.

Concluding Reflections on Indigenous Self-determination as Embodied Governance

We cannot build strong, and politically and culturally vibrant communities if we experience devastating illness. For Indigenous birth workers, birth is an act of resurgence. Birth is an act of love for our people, love for the Land that raised us, and love for the Water that brought us forth. Birth is a process binding us to one another in relationship and accountability. Birth is what connects us to our ancestors before us and to our generations to come. Birth does not begin with conception, nor does it end at entry into this world. Birth begins in the Spirit World and continues through the entire life of the being.

In our roles as students, instructors, researchers, community members, and relatives, we aspire to situate our work in a broader context of interconnected efforts toward building strong and healthy Indigenous Nations. We hope to use our work to challenge current narratives on Indigenous cultural, spiritual, and political perspectives, as well as to broaden theoretical models of governance through Indigenous conceptions of relationship, regeneration, and resurgence. There are wellsprings of hope and strength throughout the country, which exemplify the centring of Indigenous healing paradigms toward resurgent Indigenous governance traditions. Whether it be community health leadership in the form of youth engagement in the Reimagining Attawapiskat project or We Matter campaign; sexual education and self-determination as demonstrated by the Native Youth Sexual Health Network in Canada or La Colectiva Feminista en Construcción in Puerto Rico; food security and Land-based sovereignty at the Dechinta Centre for Research and Learning, Northwest Territories; or Indigenous-led approaches to birthing practice and childcare at Seventh Generation Midwives Toronto: these are all sources of new learning, healing, regeneration, and understanding.[2]

This advancement in knowledge and awareness demonstrates how although all genders carry responsibilities for the reproduction of cultural knowledge for future generations, women are uniquely positioned as leaders with the capacity not only to infuse cultural and spiritual realms with political meaning, but also to connect political governance models with gendered healing and wellness traditions. As a Cheyenne proverb states, "A nation is not conquered until the hearts of women are on the ground" (qtd. in Lavell-Harvard and Corbiere Lavell vii). Going further, this chapter has highlighted how as long as the hearts of women are intimately connected to the Land and Water, they will pursue Indigenous political consciousness through embodied governance as enacted sovereignty. Embodied governance relations extend out from the Land through bodies and into the webs of relational experience to and with one another as kin, allies, and community members. Million reminds us that in this way "the nurturing inclusiveness that is often modelled as an ideal in kinship teaches us that we form one another and create social and spiritual relations that we extend and that are extended to us in radiating bursts of affective interrelations that also include nonhuman relations" (180). Through situating our bodies as sites of governance, the very breath that moves through our bodies is a life force connecting our independent enactments of sovereignty and story into larger constellations of interbeing, relationship, and interconnectivity. In a similar vein, as Kānaka Maoli scholar Noelani Goodyear-Kaʻōpua shares: "Ea refers to political independence and is often translated as 'sovereignty,' life, breath, among other things. A shared characteristic in each of these translations is that ea is an active state of being. Like breathing, ea cannot be achieved or possessed; it requires constant action day after day, generation after generation. It extends back to the birth of the land itself"; it is a "word that describes emergence, such as volcanic islands from the depths of the ocean," and refers to "political independence as well as life itself" (4). What are the ways that we can understand ea in our own languages, cultures, and teachings? A prayer sent to Erynne by her elder and Great Uncle Ted Chartrand says Ayis Kihewini Pimatisiwin, Your (Creator) breath is life. Ea, as breath, Yehewini as breath, the animation of our bodies through spirit, life and relationship within a framework of political emancipation and wellness encodes different meanings and imaginaries of the boundaries between personal and political. The very fact that our "our lands are in fact living ancestors" situates power, energy, and force derived from the Land as something very "distinct from Western iterations of sovereignty specifically because of the continuous renewal of land-based, familial relationships requiring mutual care" (Goodyear-Kaʻōpua et al. 22). Ea the breath, or in Cree-Michif, *Yehewini Pimatisiwin,* Breath of Life, animates our personal expressions of creative agency, determination, and embodied governance in a relational praxis of sovereignty. Embodied governance, Land as body and body as Land, upholds and protects cultural knowledge; it promotes pathways to cultivate decolonial possibilities for healing and wellness grounded within healthy vibrant families, communities, and sovereign Nations.

Endnotes

1 The words Land and Water are capitalized because our teachings tell us that Land and Water are sovereign entities of their own (just as we would capitalize a country or name of a person), and both entities comprise territory.

2 Native Youth Sexual Health Network is an organization by and for Indigenous youth that works across issues of sexual and reproductive health, rights and justice throughout the United States and Canada (www.nativeyouthsexualhealthnetwork.com). The Dechinta Centre for Research and Learning is a northern-led initiative delivering Land-based, university credited educational experiences led by northern leaders, experts, elders, and professors to engage northern and southern youth in a transformative curricula based on the cutting-edge needs of Canada's North (http://dechinta.ca/). Seventh Generation Midwives is a group of primary caregivers who provide high-quality maternity care to women and their families from the City of Toronto, particularly those from the downtown area, and from the Aboriginal community (http://www.sgmt.ca/).

Works Cited

Adelson, N. "The Embodiment of Inequity: Health Disparities in Aboriginal Canada." *Canadian Journal of Public Health*, vol. 96, no. 2, 2005, pp. S45-S61.

Alfred, Taiaiake. *Wasáse: Indigenous Pathways of Action and Freedom.* University of Toronto Press, 2005.

Anderson, Kim. *A Recognition of Being: Reconstructing Native Womanhood.* Sumach Press, 2000.

Altamirano-Jiménez, Isabel. *Indigenous Encounters with Neoliberalism: Place, Women and the Environment in Canada and Mexico.* University of British Columbia Press, 2013.

Atleo, Richard. *Tsawalk: A Nuu-chah-nulth Worldview.* Universit of British Columbia Press, 2004.

Bellrichard, Chantelle. "Bringing Birth Back to Temote Manitoba First Nation: Women from Norway House Refusing to Leave for Delivery." CBC News, 2014, www.cbc.ca/news/indigenous/bringing-birth-back-to-remote-manitoba-first-nation-1.2703154. Accessed 20 July 2018.

Casumbal-Salazar, Iokepa. "A Fictive Kinship- Making "Modernity," "Ancient Hawaiians," and the Telescopes on Mauna Kea." *Native American and Indigenous Studies*, vol. 4, no. 2, 2017, pp. 1-30.

Chad et al. "In Their Own Words: First Nations Girls' Resilience as Reflected Through their Undersatndings of Health." *Pimatisiwin: A Journal of Aboriginal and Indigenous Community Health*, vol. 11, no. 1, 2013, pp. 1-15.

Chandler, MJ, and CE Lalonde. "Folk Theories of Mind and Self: A Cross-Cultural Study of Suicide in Native and Non-Native Groups." *The Development of Theories of Mind and the Construction of Cognitive Abilities*, edited by A Marchetti and O Sempio Milano, Franco Angeli, 1994.

Chilisa, Bagele. *Indigenous Research Methodologies.* Sage Publications, 2011.

Corntassel, Jeff. "We Belong to Each Other: Resurgent Indigenous Nations." *Manatake*, 2013,www.manataka.org/page2661.html. Accessed 20 July 2018.

Corntassel Jeff, et al. "Everyday Acts of Resurgence: People Places Practices." *International Cry*, 2018, intercontinentalcry.org/everyday-acts-resurgence-people-places-practices/. Accessed 7 Aug. 2018:

Coulthard, Glen. "Place against Empire: Understanding Indigenous Anti- Colonialism." *Affinities: A Journal of Radical Theory, Culture, and Action*, vol. 4, 2010, pp. 79-83.

Fanon, Frantz. *Black Skin White Masks.* Grove Press, 1967.

Gomes, T.A.,Young Leon, and L.Brown. "Indigenous Health Leadership: Protocols, Policy, and Practice." *Pimatisiwin: A Journal of Aboriginal and Indigenous Community Health* Vol. 11, no. 3, 2013, pp. 565-78.

Goodyear-Ka'opua, Noelani et al. *A Nation Rising: Hawaiian Movements for Life, Land and Sovereignty.* Duke University Press, 2014.

Halseth, Regine. Aboriginal Women in Canada: Gender, Socio Economic Determinants of *Health and Initiatives to Close the Wellness Gap. National Collaborating Centre for Aboriginal Health.* National Collaborating Centre for Aboriginal Health, 2013.

Hancock, Robert. "'We Know Who Are Relatives Are': Métis Identities in Historical, Political and Legal Contexts." *Calling Our Families Home: Métis Peoples' Experiences with Child Welfare*, edited by Jeannine Carriere and Catherine Richardson, Charlton Publishing, 2017, pp. 9-30.

Health Canada. "First Nations and Inuit Health Branch In-House Statistics." Canadian Vital Statistics Death Database. *Statistics Canada*, 2010. www.canada.ca/en/indigenous-services-canada/services/first-nations-inuit-health/reports-publications/aboriginal-health-research/statistical-profile-health-first-nations-canada-vital-statistics-atlantic-western-canada-2001-2002-health-canada-2011.html. Accessed 20 July 2018.

Hoover, Elizabeth, et al. "Indigenous Peoples of North America: Environmental Exposures and Reproductive Justice." *Environmental Health Perspectives*, vol. 120, no. 2, 2012, pp. 1645-49.

Kirmayer, Laurence, and Gail Guthrie Valaskakis, editors. *Healing Traditions: The Mental Health of Aboriginal Peoples in Canada*. UBC Press, 2009.

Kovach, Margaret. *Indigenous Methodologies: Characteristics, Conversations and Contexts*. University of Toronto Press, 2009.

Kuokkanen, Rauna. "Gendered Violence and Politics in Indigenous Communities." *International Feminist Journal of Politics*, vol. 17, no.2, 2014, pp. 271-88.

Ladner, Kiera L. "Understanding the Impact of Self-Determination on Communities Crisis."

National Aboriginal Health Organization (NAHO) 2009. URL no longer available. Accessed January 2014.

Leyland Andrew, et al. *Health and Health Care Implications of Systemic Racism on Indigenous Peoples in Canada*. Prepared by the Indigenous Health Working Group of the College of Family Physicians of Canada and Indigenous Physicians Association of Canada. The College of Family Physicians of Canada, 2016.

Loppie Charlotte, et al. "Aboriginal Experiences with Racism and its Impacts." Social Determinants of Health. *National Collaborating Centre for Aboriginal Health (NCCAH)*, 2014. www.ccnsa-nccah.ca/docs/determinants/FS-AboriginalExperiencesRacismImpacts-Loppie-Reading-deLeeuw-EN.pdf. Accessed 3 Aug. 2018.

Lavell-Harvard, D. Memee and Jeanette Corbiere Lavell, editors. *Until our Hearts are on the Ground: Aboriginal Mothering, Oppression, Resistance and Rebirth*. Demeter Press, 2006.

Manuel, George and Michael Posluns. *The Fourth World: An Indian Reality*. Free Press, 1974.

McCormick, R. "Healing through Interdependence: The Role of Connecting in First Nations Healing Practices." Canadian Journal of Counselling, vol. 31, no. 3, 1997, pp. 172-84.

Million, D. *Therapeutic Nations: Healing in an Age of Indigenous Human Rights.* The University of Arizona University Press, 2013.

Mundel, E, and G. Chapman. "A Decolonizing Approach to Health Promotion in Canada: The Case of the Urban Aboriginal Community Kitchen Garden Project." *Health Promotion International*, vol. 25, no. 2, 2010, pp. 166-73.

Native Women's Association of Canada (NWAC). "Aboriginal Women and Health Care in Canada. *NWAC*, 2002. www.nwac.ca/wp-content/uploads/2015/05/2007-Social-Determinants-of-Health-and-Canada%E2%80%99s-Aboriginal-Women-NWAC-Submission-to-WHO-Commission.pdf. Accessed 3 Aug. 2018.

Native Youth Sexual Health Network (NYSHN). Report. "NYSHN Statement to National Energy Board Regarding Line 9 Pipeline Proposal." *NYSHN*, 2013. www.nativeyouthsexualhealth.com/pressreleases.html, Accessed 7 Aug. 2018.

Reading, Charlotte. *Policies, Programs and Strategies to Address Aboriginal Racism: A Canadian Perspective.* Social Determinants of Health. National Collaborating Centre for Aboriginal Health (NCCAH), 2014.

Reimagining Attawapiskat: Collaborative Mixed Media Storytelling Project. *Reimagining Attawapiskat*, www.reimaginingattawapiskat.com/about-reimagining-attawapiskat. Accessed 20 July 2018.

Royal Commission on Aboriginal Peoples (RCAP). *Bridging the Cultural Divide: A Report on Aboriginal People and Criminal Justice in Canada. Government of Canada*, 1996, www.bac-lac.gc.ca/eng/discover/aboriginal-heritage/royal-commission-aboriginal-peoples/Pages/item.aspx?IdNumber=517. Accessed 20 July 2018.

Simpson, Leanne. *Dancing on Our Turtle's Back.* Arbeiter Ring Press, 2011.

Smith, Linda Tuhiwai. *Decolonizing Methodologies: Research and Indigenous Peoples.* Zed Books, 2012.

Statistics Canada. *Census of Canada analytical documents: Aboriginal Peoples in Canada: First Nations People, Métis and Inuit, 2011 National Household Survey. Government of Canada*, 2011, Stout, Madeleine Dion. *Aboriginal Women's Health Research: Synthesis Project.* Centres of Excellence for Women's Health (Canada), 2001.

Sunseri, Lina. *Being Again of One Mind: Oneida Women and the Struggle for Decolonization*. University of British Columbia Press, 2011.

Suzack, Cheryl et al. *Indigenous Women and Feminism: Politics, Activism, Culture*. Universiity of British Columbia Press, 2011.

Tagalik, Shirley. *Inuit Qaujimajatuqangit: The Role of Indigenous Knowledge in Supporting Wellness in Inuit Communities in Nunavut*. Child and Youth: National Collaborating Centre for Aboriginal Health (NAHO), 2010.

Varcoe, C., et al. "Help Bring Back the Celebration of Life: A Community-Based Participatory Study of Rural Aboriginal Women's Maternity Experiences and Outcomes." *BMC Pregnancy Childbirth*, vol. 13, no. 26, 2001.

Wiebe, Sarah Marie. *Everyday Exposure: Indigenous Mobilization and Environmental Justice in Canada's Chemical Valley*. University of British Columbia Press, 2016.

Wilson, Shawn. *Research Is Ceremony: Indigenous Research Methods*. Winnipeg: Fernwood Publishing. 2009.

Chapter Eight

Indeterminate Life: Dealing with Radioactive Contamination as a Voluntary Evacuee Mother

Maxime Polleri

On 11 March 2011, Japan experienced the most powerful earthquake ever recorded on the Japanese archipelago, followed by an equally devastating tsunami. These two successive natural disasters greatly damaged the Fukushima Daiichi Nuclear Power Plant. Subsequent human errors contributed to the nuclear meltdown of some of the power plant's reactors, causing the discharge of radioactive materials and the forced evacuation of residents within a twenty-kilometre radius. Many more individuals living beyond this officially restricted zone fled through their own initiative—putting the number of evacuees at more than 160,000. In the following years, members of the local and central government have repeatedly stated that the levels of radiation released during the disaster were too low to pose any major adverse health effects to the population of Japan. The same officials were also quick to assert that the more serious source of harm to the affected public would be the resultant psychological fear linked with radiation.

These historical facts are known by many, yet they only tell one version of the story. Indeed, there is another parallel experience running alongside this official narrative—namely, the often unheard story of the individuals living in the shadow of these sanctioned statistics, which constitute the official understanding of what is now known as the Fukushima nuclear disaster.

Fast forward to 11 March 2016. Five years have passed since the disaster, and I am listening to a speech being given by Akiko Uno, the founder of the National Refugee Association. Mrs. Uno, a voluntary evacuee (*jishu hinansha*) from Fukushima, did not fall within the official evacuation perimeter. Fearing radioactive contamination nonetheless, she formed a group of mothers seeking the right to officially evacuate from an environment they consider harmful to themselves and their children. In front of a full audience, she invites these mothers to share their experiences as voluntary evacuees. Many go on to voice their concerns about the hardships of rationalizing the presence of an imperceptible harm—radioactive contamination—and about the apparent increase of thyroid cancers in children, which they believe is linked to radiation exposure. At one point, a young mother suddenly bursts into tears. The only sounds heard are the woman's sobs and the constant electrical whine of the microphone. Thus, even as government officials contend that concerns about radioactive contamination are unwarranted, the story of that young mother, convulsing with tears, points toward a different set of experiences.

In this chapter, I explore how Japanese mothers who have chosen to evacuate of their own free will embody radioactive hazards resulting from the Fukushima disaster. As an anthropologist, I explore the notion of embodiment as the lived experience of radioactive hazards, constituted through corporeal knowledge and affective entanglements, and located within specific sociocultural, gendered, and technological contexts. Employing an ethnographical approach, I follow the story of one voluntary evacuee, a mother named Noriko Matsumoto, whose experience forms the primary analytical framework of this chapter.[1] I offer a different narrative from the one presented by government officials—an alternative story that exemplifies how voluntary evacuee mothers resist, in part, the official safety discourse that downplays the risk of radioactive contamination for specific actors. At the same time, I show how these mothers' efforts to resist the official narrative of safety produce alternative ways of articulating their lives. My data were collected through ongoing interviews with Noriko, as well as participant observation of her ongoing attempts to rationalize and express the potential threats engendered by radioactive contamination. In a context of widespread anxiety brought on by radioactive contaminants, I argue that life has become an indeterminate locus for these mothers—oscillating between an uncertain past and an unfamiliar future while destabilizing social and corporal boundaries. This has forced these individuals to constantly reconfigure their identities (particularly their identities as mothers).

To theoretically explore the entangled relationships between radioactive contamination and a mother's experience, I draw from the material-discursive framework of feminist theorist Karen Barad, who has developed the concept of "agential realism." Through this concept, Barad argues for a new framework that ties together epistemological and ontological issues. She notes that realism is "not about representations of an independent reality, but about the real consequences, interventions, creative possibilities, and responsibilities of intraacting within the world" (188). Avoiding the word "interacting," as it presupposes that two preexisting entities interact, Barad instead uses the word "intra-action" to refer to the "be-in," where the matter and meaning meet (179). In this understanding, subjects and objects are no longer determined prior to their interaction. Barad's viewpoint privileges neither the material nor the cultural realm per se, but rather the mutual constitution of entangled agencies. Accordingly, this chapter does not view radioactive contamination as a fixed entity defined by a single body of experts who hold the yardstick of truth about nature. Rather, as per agential realism, it grounds and situates knowledge claims in local experiences—and Noriko's understanding of radiation is closely related to her own life experience both as an individual and as a mother. Indeed, agential realism mediates between the materiality that radioactive contamination embodies and the symbolism that it takes on in a specific local environment.

Radioactive Contamination: Background and Current Literature

During the Fukushima nuclear disaster, radioactive contaminants (i.e., radionuclides, including iodine131, cesium134, and cesium137) scattered across Japan, and potentially subjected citizens to internal and/or external radiation exposure.[2] These radionuclides produce ionizing radiation, which can sever the chemical bonds in the cells of living beings and damage DNA, the molecules that carry biological information. In trying to repair themselves, cells can make mistakes in the form of errors in the DNA blueprint (Sakiyama). The subsequent mutation (i.e., a permanent alteration of the cell's reproductive outcomes) can result in somatic effects (e.g., cancers occurring in the bodies of exposed individuals), and/or in transgenerational effects (i.e., mutations present in the egg or sperm germ cells of exposed individuals, which can potentially be transmitted to future generations). Above a certain level of exposure (namely, one hundred millisieverts a year), radiation is known to "impair immunity to infection and increase the risk of leukaemia, certain sorts of solid cancers, cataracts and probably also heart disease and stroke" (Morris-Suzuki 336).

Still, there is no clear consensus regarding the health effects of long-term, low-level chronic exposure to radiation, which is what many of the citizens of Japan are living with. In general, the field of radiological protection adopts a linear nonthreshold hypothesis deeming risk to be proportional to level of exposure. The real picture, however, is more complex than that. As Tessa Morris-Suzuki states, "All experts agree that the impact varies greatly per type of radiation, the nature of the radioactive substances involved, the age and gender of those exposed, and the nature of the exposure" (336).

In the case of a nuclear disaster, evacuation measures are based on a risk-benefit analysis, which considers the number of people who may be harmed if they were to remain in the affected area. Partly based on the recommendations of the International Commission on Radiological Protection, the Japanese state has, in the aftermath of the Fukushima disaster, subsequently increased the permissible exposure rate (i.e., the mandatory evacuation trigger) from one millisievert to twenty millisieverts. This new threshold has been criticized by members of the impacted population, such as mothers and medical doctors, as representing a concession to economic and political imperatives (Polleri). To monitor the long-term health effects of the radioactive contamination related to the Fukushima nuclear disaster, an epidemiological study (the Fukushima Prefecture Health Management Survey) was launched by Japan's national government. The senior director of this research, Shun'ichi Yamashita, was quick to state that the levels of radiation were too low to pose any health effects to the local population and that the real harm would be psychological. Perhaps best known for his (in)famous reflection that "If one laughs, then radiation is not scary" (*warate ireba hōshanō ha kowakunai*), Shun'ichi Yamashita was a hated figure among the mothers I interviewed.[3]

There are, of course, many complex issues involved in regards to the government's official threshold of risk—issues going well beyond the scope of this chapter (see Morris-Suzuki). For instance, many other studies have already pinpointed the actual mitigation of the risk in a "state that seeks to manage the crisis according to its own agenda" (Slater et al. 486). In a context of so much scientific uncertainty, an emerging body of work is dedicated to capturing the (un)official experiences of the people living through the Fukushima disaster. These studies include in-depth ethnographies of how Japanese mothers experience the resultant radioactive contamination. In one study of food and citizen science, Nicolas Sternsdorff-Cisterna demonstrates that many mothers create alternative scientific spaces to deal with radiation risk. In the same vein, Aya Hirata Kimura has focused on the techno-scientific enterprise of mothers attempting to test food for radioactive contamination, and has pinpointed the stiff social sanctions they face while doing so. David Slater et al. highlight similar concerns—namely, that mothers expressing fears about radiation are seen to be challenging the normative societal roles and gendered responsibilities of Japanese women and are thereby discredited. Rika Morioka indirectly tackles similar issues by highlighting how the construction of Japanese masculinity impedes mothers from easily articulating their concerns. Together, these works contribute to the anthropological literature about radioactive risk by showing how risk perception is rooted in local knowledge, cultural understanding of the environment, and gendered affective feelings. Notably, these studies' findings illustrate the importance of different social contexts in terms of rationalizing scientific uncertainty.

The current chapter contributes to this body of scholarship by focusing on voluntary evacuee mothers in particular. Yet rather than peering through a lens of risk subjectivity or scientific uncertainty to explore the disorientation and alienation radioactive contamination has brought to these mothers' lives, it takes an alternative path by focusing on indeterminacy. As Morris-Suzuki explains, "'Risk' exists where an event may or may not occur, but the odds of its occurring are relatively well known; 'uncertainty' is the situation where the broad parameters of a risk are understood but science is not (or not yet) capable of accurately assessing the odds" (349). However, with both risk and uncertainty, there remains a clear distinction between human agency and radioactive contamination. Indeed, the notion of indeterminacy goes beyond risk and uncertainty, as it emphasizes "the human-nature interaction that lies at the heart of issues like ... radiation releases" (Morris-Suzuki 349-50). Astrid Schrader further contributes to this point: "The very idea of an epistemological uncertainty presupposes an a priori separation of the epistemological question of 'how we know' from the ontological status of 'what we know,' where only the former, that is, our knowledge is allowed to vary" (277). Consequently, she argues for a move away from "epistemological uncertainties to ontological indeterminacies," and claims uncertainties "assume the possibility of certainties as horizon or telos, and therefore the possibility of their removal" (275-80).

For voluntary evacuee mothers in postdisaster Japan, radioactive contamination has resulted in just that: a total upheaval of their horizons as mothers. Indeed, when life as they formerly understood it has mutated beyond current comprehension and understanding, notions of risk and uncertainty are not the best operative modalities for making sense of radioactive contamination. As such, I argue that voluntary evacuee mothers maintain an inherently indeterminate relationship with radiation itself and that this relationship must be constantly reconfigured in a new reality where nothing is fixed in advance.

Noriko's Story

"There's a giant incinerator burning decontamination waste near my home in Fukushima.... Ashes are falling on people's clothes, and when I made my concerns known to the local officials, I was told that I shouldn't worry, as they use special filters.... But honestly, how can you live in such conditions?" That's how Noriko Matsumoto ends our conversation in a small coffee shop near downtown Shinjuku. She no longer has the energy she initially had at the beginning of our interview, two hours earlier. Her brown eyes seem lost in a not-so-distant past; perhaps she is pondering the many changes radioactive contamination has brought into her life during the past number of years.

When the disaster happened, Noriko was living in the city of Koriyama, situated within the prefecture of Fukushima. Koriyama was not included in the mandatory evacuation zone, but Noriko was so concerned about radioactive contamination that in the immediate aftermath of the disaster, she flew to Tokyo with her daughter. A couple of months later, she decided to return to Fukushima, as she believed the situation had settled. As she explains to me: "Of course ... I was still worried about radiation. But in those days, I heard Dr. Yamashita, a well-known specialist on radiation exposure from Nagasaki, saying repeatedly that it was safe in Fukushima and that no health effects would appear." Temporarily appeased by this rhetoric, Noriko brought her daughter back to Koriyama to resume school. However, her daughter soon began to suffer from diarrhea, nausea, and recurrent nosebleeds during which the blood had "a very dark and unusual colour." Children of her work colleagues were suffering from similar ailments, and these symptoms began to implant a seed of doubt in Noriko's mind.

Spurred on by her growing anxiety, Noriko began a journey of self-erudition; she read everything she could find about the potential side effects of radioactive contamination. She even borrowed a Geiger counter from the city office to measure the radiation in her house: "Outside of our home, the radiation level peaked at around 2.7 microsieverts per hour. I did not know what those numbers meant at first, but when I searched on the Internet, I discovered that this was quite abnormal!" Alarmed by this new information, Noriko and her daughter left Fukushima to stay with Noriko's sister in Tokyo.

As voluntary evacuees, however, they received little recognition from the state and were put on a waiting list for access to temporary apartments. After many months of waiting, they were finally assigned an apartment in Kawasaki, but her daughter was already enrolled in a junior high school in Tokyo. Noriko's husband, meanwhile, remained in Fukushima for his work, and they could be together as a family only once every few months. In this way, the radioactive contaminants released during the disaster were not Fukushima's only unstable by-products; as Noriko notes "Our family has also become fragmented" (*bara bara*). Within this context, radioactive contamination brought indeterminacy into the social roles Noriko used to view as inseparable not so long ago: those of wife and mother. Indeed, in terms of the idealized traditional role of Japanese women, the ubiquitous phrase "Good Wife, Wise Mother" has long set the recurrent pattern of gendered relationships (Slater et al.). Yet biological concerns linked with radioactive contamination are now subsuming traditional assumptions and bringing, as Slater et al. argue, a "potential conflict between the two roles that young women are expected to fulfill" (496).

Two years after the disaster, Noriko became sick with Reiter syndrome, a form of collagen disease. As Noriko notes, "Usually, it's supposed to leave after one year, but I still haven't recovered from it yet, and it's been more than three years." She goes on to tell me that there are three known reasons why this illness occurs, but none of the tests she undertook could identify the actual cause of the disease in her particular case. As such, she can only explain the source of her illness through radiation exposure: "When people think about radioactive exposure, the first thing that comes to their mind is cancer. But there's much more than that ... [With low doses] you don't die right away. It brings a lot of small problems." Although high doses of radiation exposure can obviously present immediate and irrefutable danger to biological life, Noriko's chronic ailments, which she perceives as being linked to low-dose radiation exposure, exemplify a different perception of radiological harm. This perception holds that radiological contamination affects not only life but also the quality of life. It is precisely this subtlety—a distinction that cannot be overstated for the affected individuals—the governmental experts just cannot grasp, according to Noriko.

Yet beyond her affliction, Noriko is much more concerned about the wellbeing of her daughter. For instance, she is anxious about the specific threat posed by radioactive iodine (iodine131)—a dangerous and short-lived by-product of fission in nuclear power plants that some link with an apparent increase in thyroid cancers among children. For that reason, in 2011, Noriko participated in the Fukushima Prefecture Health Management Survey to receive information about her and her daughter's overall radiation exposure following the disaster. However, "We have never received any data whatsoever," claims Noriko. "They didn't contact us with details; [they] simply told us that it was OK."

Furthermore, Noriko is not satisfied with how the survey determined exposure levels. To calculate their initial dose of external exposure, the survey asked Noriko and her daughter to itinerate their displacements in the aftermath of the disaster. Thus, their exposure level was calculated based on their recollections of their movements following the disaster. For Noriko, there is nothing empirical or scientific in this process. "Calculating [based] on your own memory is not enough," she tells me angrily. "Especially for evacuees who might not remember the whole sequence of events clearly!" As a result, Noriko now believes their real dose of external exposure will never be known.[4] She finds this upsetting, for even though external exposure means that the radiation passes through the body without remaining inside of it, the potential for genetic damage remains.

Overall, Noriko feels she and her daughter have been unnecessarily exposed to radiation. She also believes the dosage estimates she received are simply inaccurate due to both the intangibility of radioactive contamination and the inefficiency of governmental responses. What's more, new data has revealed the state initially underestimated the spread of the radioactive plume. As Noriko laments, "Now we know that the radiation level in Koriyama was quite high after March 15. If we had been given accurate information from our government, I would not have made my daughter come back. I truly regret what I did."

In Noriko's narrative, the original exposure and its subsequent damage remain unknown. In her case, radiation affirms an "indeterminate relationship between being and becoming and between 'past' and 'future'" (Schrader 278). Indeed, for Noriko, the link between the past and the future is no longer "associated with what is already given or known"; rather, it has become "a matter of inheritance to which not only humans contribute" (Schrader 299). The risk communication strategy adopted by the Japanese authorities, however, contradicts such indeterminacy and remains inapplicable to how Noriko experiences radioactive contamination, both as an individual and as a mother. As Robert Paine argues, "The very notion of risk introduces options.... Risk, then, pertains to probability calculations about danger and, hence, to the 'cost' of a projected undertaking" (68). For Noriko, radioactive contamination itself is precisely the variable that's blurring this capacity for calculation. As she explains: "When you're sick from the flu, you know that your sickness is coming from there, but not with radiation. You don't get sick right away; you might not even be sure of the real cause. Even the experts can't know for sure."

For Noriko, probability calculations are inapplicable to the situation in which she and her daughter are now living. Like the stochastic process surrounding radioactive damage, her life is filled with unpredictable transformations due to the influence of random variables over which she feels a lack of control. For instance, referring to the apparent increase in thyroid cancer among children, Noriko remarks, "What option do children have against that?" Ironically, the thyroid is the endocrine gland enabling the growth of children, which is symbolically what many Fukushima mothers feel deprived of: the possibility of a bright future that will allow their children to flourish. Radiation, therefore, creates an impossible situation—namely, a state of not knowing whether one's (future) symptoms are linked to exposure. This feeling of doubt is precisely what cast Noriko in the role of carrying an agonizing burden, which is now part of her daily life.

Countermeasures

Dissatisfied with the state's approach toward radioactive contamination and pushed by a maternal will to adequately protect her daughter, Noriko began to look for others who shared similar concerns. Through contacts, she discovered the organization *Datsu hibaku jitsugen netto* (Network to Evacuate People from Radiation), which is how I initially met her. The organization had formerly supported a legal case filed on behalf of several children who needed a court to rule in favour of their being evacuated. After the failure of this legal proceeding, however, the group diversified its mandate. Noriko had become an active member in this organization, and for one of our first meetings, I follow her during an antinuclear demonstration held in Shinjuku.

For more than two hours, Noriko walks alongside her fellow activists, who are criticizing what they refer to as "the safety campaign" (i.e., the attempts of the government to downplay the health effects of radiation exposure). Tirelessly, they shout slogans such as "Let the children escape from Fukushima!" and "We won't be silenced by the government!" The group's main point of contention is the maximum threshold for permissible exposure, which has been increased from one millisievert to twenty millisieverts. Not far from me, an elderly female protester shouts, "Professionals in the radio-medical domain are not allowed to receive a dose that is higher than 0.2 millisieverts, but mothers and children can live in an area of twenty millisieverts? What is wrong with Japan!?"

As the demonstration approaches the commercial district of Shinjuku, the rallying cries of the group are drowned out by the popular music emanating from the giant sound systems of nearby shopping centres. Noriko's hand-written sign is suddenly dwarfed by the twenty-foot-tall electronic billboards dominating the streets. At the end of the demonstration, everyone shakes hands and goes their own ways. The activists, who were not so long ago criticizing the government, return to being regular people—just mothers minding their own business. Being an activist and a refugee is a difficult task to keep up on a daily basis, it seems. Indeed, as Noriko tells me, "You need a good balance between your life and your activism." Finding such balance is a never-ending process, and as with radioactive contamination itself, the role Noriko embodies (i.e., wife, mother, citizen activist) remains indeterminate.

Apart from demonstrations, the organization runs regular workshops where members meet to discuss their situations. Most presentations take place in a small basement, which is always packed. During these meetings, mothers deliberate over the current state of radioactive contamination. They speak about the types of food most prone to radioactive contamination and that thereby should be avoided, such as mushrooms, green leafy vegetables, and *yuzu* (a sort of Japanese citrus). They even discuss the toxicity of specific radionuclides and their effects on the different sexes. The way these mothers critically evaluate radiation exposure represents a sharp contrast to the official narrative, which treats "residents with high sensitivity to radiation (including pregnant women and infants) the same as professional radiation workers" (Fukushima Booklet Publication Committee 14), especially in light of the raised exposure threshold (to twenty millisieverts). Mothers such as Noriko find it impossible to condone the fact that their own government made this decision.

In this way, radioactive contamination also epitomizes the change in the relationship mothers, as citizens, maintain with the Japanese state. This relationship between citizens and the state is now catalyzed and mediated by the acquisition of a scientific expertise—what Sternsdorff-Cisterna calls a "scientific citizenship." Voluntary evacuee mothers could stereotypically be thought of as putting forward sentimental speeches. As already emphasized, however, this couldn't be further from the truth, as they first and foremost mobilize a scientific discourse about radioactive contamination—a discourse that subsequently allows them to criticize the decisions taken by their very own government.

Yet just as Noriko was slowly adjusting to this new life, the government announced that financial help for voluntary evacuees would end in March 2017. Such a policy leaves many voluntary evacuee mothers with no choice but to return to Fukushima. As with other mothers, Noriko is critical of the governmental revitalization projects (*fukkō*) that aim to repatriate citizens to their former hometown: "All I see on TV are ads about revitalization, but they don't mean anything for us." In the years that have passed since Noriko's evacuation, her daughter, who was originally an elementary student, has become a young woman; she is already accustomed to a new life, and there is no point in her going back to an environment that would expose them, in Noriko's view, to chronic low-dose radiation. Indeed, for Noriko, radiation damage leaves an unwanted legacy for children such as her daughter, who are forced to bear a responsibility that should not be theirs. In an attempt to change this situation, and in sharp contrast to the government-sponsored revitalization process, Noriko is looking to create a new legacy for her daughter. Specifically, she aims to achieve this legacy through the creation of a diary (*techō*) that can relate one's personal history of exposure and sickness.

I follow Noriko to the Big Pallet Fukushima Conference Centre, where an assembly for the creation of an irradiation booklet is being established. Interestingly, a survivor from the Hiroshima nuclear bombing, an elderly woman named Eiko Ono, is also present at the assembly. As an irradiated survivor (*hibakusha*), Mrs. Ono is in possession of an "Abomb survivor health notebook" (*hibakusha kenkō techō*). This notebook certifies that Mrs. Ono was indeed a victim of the bombing, and, as such, guarantees government coverage of her medical fees in case of illness. Mrs. Ono believes that many of her illnesses are linked to her original radiation exposure, and she encourages the mothers present at the assembly to begin tracking their displacements and health histories as soon as possible. She explains that the notebook has relieved many of her worries about financial matters, and she is highly in favour of the creation of a similar handbook for residents of Fukushima.

Noriko agrees that the evacuees from Fukushima need something similar. "I believe that this is absolutely necessary, and I want that for my daughter!" she says. Indeed, such a handbook would stand as an individual record, a personal archive, that could act as a countermeasure to the official state chronicles. Importantly, the mere advocacy for these handbooks highlights the fact that many voluntary evacuee mothers are now experiencing the threat of radioactive contamination as a form of financial precarity, particularly in light of potential medical costs.

The need for medical follow up and health intervention is facing increasing criticism, however, not only from the government, but also from other Fukushima residents. As Noriko claims: "There are a lot of old people who refuse to believe information that doesn't appear on television. It's very hard to convince them. They tell us things like 'The country is saying that it's safe, so why do you contradict them?' Mothers who criticize how the Fukushima disaster is being handled are being called unpatriotic and selfish." In this context, an integral part of motherhood (i.e., mothers worrying about the long-term wellbeing of their children) is becoming an act of selfishness and antipatriotism. In Noriko's view, however, voluntary evacuee mothers work for the common good; after all, she sees the government's revitalization policies as supporting the state's economic interests rather than the citizens' interests. In her words, "The government is constantly repeating the slogan of 'recovery and reconstruction,' and in doing so they encourage voluntary evacuees to return to areas of high risk." For these mothers, then, radioactive contamination has gone well beyond biology per se, and is now understood as a form of structural injustice perpetrated by the state against its citizens.

Discussion

Today, in Fukushima, radioactive contamination is part of people's everyday lives. Air dose measurers, which display the current level of radiation in the air, are found across the prefecture to help residents assess the risk of radiation exposure. Every time Noriko returns to Fukushima to see her husband, however, these machines become more than mere tools in her mind—they are reminders that the disaster is still happening. For instance, when the levels are too high, parents forbid their children from playing outside. In such ways, mothers do all they can to protect their children in this normalized state of emergency—even as they are agonizingly aware of how short they are falling in their efforts. Indeed, the word *migoroshi* (which can be translated as "letting someone die") was frequently uttered by the mothers I interviewed; such echoes of Foucault's biopower—the prerogative of a nation-state to make live and let die—was clearly discernable amid Noriko's narrative, too. With so much at stake, these voluntary evacuee mothers have felt forced to relegate their traditional gendered roles, not to mention the stability of a household and financial security, to second-rank priorities.

Yet beyond health matters per se, these voluntary evacuee mothers also experience postdisaster radiation exposure through processes of structural injustice and disparities in values between the lived reality of the evacuees and the revitalization projects of the nation-state. Although the local and national governments have repeatedly argued that worrying about radiation exposure is unnecessary for these residents, Noriko's experience demonstrates that mutual exclusion between radiation exposure and one's life is simply impossible. Radioactive contamination does not exist as an absolute entity; it remains distinct only in relation to its "mutual constitution" (Barad) through individuals such as Noriko. And the relationship Noriko maintains with radiation does not itself remain fixed or finite. Instead, it is constantly being (re)negotiated, as exemplified through her experiences. As such, radioactive contamination is not a question of risk probability for mothers, as this posits a stable ontology (i.e., a given state of being upon which a calculated action leads to a rational choice). Rather, radiation has changed precisely what these mothers used to take for granted, bringing them into a world that requires new modes of feeling and perception.

Indeed, radiation puts forward a set of questions that people usually never have to think about: how do I wash my children's clothes, will the washer become contaminated? As another young mother from Fukushima articulates:

> I'm always thinking about radiation. Is there some radioactivity on those flowers? Can I let my baby touch them? Now it might be fine, but what about a decade from now? Children can't protect themselves; they can't play outside or go out. They can't do anything, and that's supposed to be what we call protection?

> I loved Fukushima so much, but now it has been sullied; we can't go out to enjoy nature as we once did.

As the narrative of this young mother exemplifies, epistemological and ontological inquiries are no longer mutually distinct. Moreover, her musings highlight a unique experience with temporality, which underscores a peculiar embodiment of radiological harm as well as the malleability of corporal boundaries.

As noted earlier, radioactive harm can involve a displacement in time, and has the potential to be genetically transferred across generations. Consequently, for worried mothers, the embodiment of radiological hazards is not merely experienced through their own corporeality, but equally through other bodies (notably their children). Moreover, for young would-be mothers living in a situation of chronic exposure, radiation hazards could equally be embodied in the idea of an unborn child. Clearly, in such situations, potential harm from radiation exposure moves beyond present concerns to take root in the future.

Consequently, radiation completely reorganizes Fukushima residents' everyday thinking, in which the present is being torn between an uncertain future and a past where the original exposure and damage remain unknown. Each of these indeterminate origins executes what Kim Fortun calls the "future anterior." As Fortun explains, "The future inhabits the present, yet it also has yet to come—rather like the way toxins inhabit the bodies of those exposed, setting up the future, but not yet manifest as disease, or even as an origin from which a specific and known disease will come" (354). The causality and responsibility surrounding the danger of radioactive contamination thereby varies within how radioactivity itself is being enacted (Schrader). In Noriko's case, she confronts and challenges the threat head on. The hardships voluntary evacuee mothers face in the aftermath of the Fukushima disaster are staggering to say the least. Although Noriko's narratives can sometimes emphasize a functionalist discourse in which individuals have little control over radioactive contamination, she has never positioned herself as a passive victim.

Paradoxically, Noriko's ever-present state of indeterminacy acts as a substratum enabling her to articulate new forms of being and acting as a mother. For instance, she actively engages in rationalizing the unwanted agency and legacy of radioactive contamination, going so far as to provide her daughter with the gift of a safe (i.e., uncontaminated) environment (*anshin kankyō purezento*). To articulate this gift, mothers such as Noriko have to become "experts" in radiation. Being a good and wise mother now means becoming experienced in an array of novel embodied practices—such as measuring radiation with a Geiger counter, participating in antinuclear demonstrations, and tracking displacements and illnesses in a health handbook. These new citizen-led understandings of radioactive contamination have subsequently laid the groundwork for new forms of being, in which self-erudition, activism, accusations of antipatriotism, and financial precarity are now part of voluntary evacuee mothers' lives. As such, these mothers potentially bring partial and limited forms of embodied knowledge to the already uncertain understanding of radiation.

Yet it is precisely these insights that can contribute toward a richer set of radiological protection measures. Unlike the state-sanctioned experts, these mothers' knowledge systems are not bounded by fixed and immovable interpretations, and, as such, they remain rather lively, contextualized, and politically relevant. Such vibrancy produces a sharp contrast against the static, perpetual, and ungendered governmental narrative that surrounds the risks of radioactive contamination in Fukushima today. These mothers do indeed have the right to ask crucial questions, such as where does the body end and where does it begin? And, more importantly, who decides such boundaries? In a locus of transgenerational mutations, the answers to such inquiries remain indeterminate, but that does not mean these voluntary evacuee mothers will stop searching for answers. As Claire Waterton and Brian Wynne argue, "When scientific risk assessment is not just uncertain but indeterminate, it logically requires public deliberation about the social needs, purposes and claimed benefits of the activities whose risks are being assessed" (96).

Conclusion

Noriko's experience highlights the fact that a clear separation between issues of epistemology and ontology rarely holds up in the real world. Her experience of radioactive contamination is one in which things figuratively and literally mutate toward other forms of being, and where matter and meaning become mutually articulated (Barad). In such a context, it is impossible to embrace an essentialist view of radioactive contamination as a fixed entity. Through the shifting materiality and symbolism of radioactive contamination, the former ontological state of this particular voluntary evacuee mother's life has become indeterminate. This shift is inseparable from the new forms of knowledge that voluntary evacuee mothers as a group have to master to navigate a life that has become completely unfamiliar. In the years since the disaster, Noriko has experienced an array of changes and has discovered new ways of articulating her life—ways that she could never have imagined. "Microsieverts" and "transgenerational effects"—once obscure terms reserved for a few scientists—are now part of a new vocabulary that Fukushima mothers must master. Without a doubt, Noriko's experience as a mother is both socially and symbolically different from what it used to be.

In truth, radioactive contamination enacts alternative approaches to traditional forms of maternal embodiment. For instance, afraid that their own breastmilk may have become a potential source of harm, many Fukushima mothers have resorted to more natural baby formula (Polleri 103). In this way, breastmilk becomes "a toxic substance, a source of life, a symbol of motherhood, or, most troublingly, all three" (Kosek 259). Perceiving childcare as the task of mothers exclusively has long been a pervasive trait in idealized Japanese normative culture. And although caring for their children is exactly what voluntary evacuee mothers are doing in the aftermath of the Fukushima disaster, their efforts are (ironically) being depicted as conflicting with state revitalization policies. Against this complex backdrop, motherhood is now manifested and embodied as a set of discordant practices and discourses clashing with the fundamental principles of Japanese social interaction, wherein harmony, cooperation, and consensus are relentlessly promoted.

In the end, mothers such as Noriko have been thrust into what I refer to as an "indeterminate life." Through such an understanding, life in postdisaster Japan becomes an indeterminate locus oscillating between an unknown past and an unfamiliar future; it destabilizes the social and corporal boundaries of mothers and thereby forces them to constantly reconfigure their identities and perceptions of motherhood. From the perspective of this constant interplay, radiation and oneself are no longer independent, but are engaged in the making of each other. In this way, bodies—that is, real bodies of irradiated flesh as well as bodies of knowledge—are "not simply situated in, or located in, particular environments. Rather 'environments' and 'bodies' are intra-actively coconstituted" (Barad qtd. in Schrader 283). This indeterminacy cannot be regarded as a fixed ontology in which life is simply messier and more chaotic and, hence, more real. Instead, it is a locus in which mothers like Noriko reconfigure their agency between the oscillation of different epistemologies and ontologies, where one single essentialist pole no longer informs and controls another. This indeterminacy forces mothers to reassess the paradigms related to wellbeing and the normative order that used to surround their lives; this is especially true in the context of radioactive contamination, in which maternal embodiment is understood through an entanglement of bodies, both physical and symbolic.

Amid the indeterminacies of radioactive contamination, the whole picture of postdisaster Fukushima can never be captured in its entirety. But even if it could be, I do not think that it should be, as the whole picture too often denies the very texture and poetry of life that such mothers as Noriko are so desperately trying to express through their own local experiences, counter narratives, tears, and seemingly never ending love for their children.

Endnotes

1 The participant's real name has been used with her approval.

2 Radioactive contamination can be external, if the body is affected by radiation from surrounding radionuclides, or internal, if radionuclides are ingested or inhaled.

3 Translation by the author.

4 Additionally, the Fukushima Prefecture Health Management Survey does not take into consideration the risk of internal exposure, which represents a separate hazard in addition to external exposure.

Works Cited

Barad, Karen. "Meeting the Universe Halfway: Realism and Social Constructivism without Contradiction." *Feminism, Science, and the Philosophy of Science*, edited by Lynn Hankinson Nelson and Jack Nelson, Springer, 1996, pp. 161-94.

Fortun, Kim. *Advocacy after Bhopal: Environmentalism, Disaster, New Global Orders*. The University of Chicago Press, 2001.

Fukushima Booklet Publication Committee. *10 Lessons from Fukushima: Reducing Risk and Protecting Communities from Nuclear Disasters*. FBPC, 2015.

Kimura, Aya Hirata. *Radiation Brain Moms and Citizen Scientists: The Gender Politics of Food Contamination after Fukushima*. Duke University Press, 2016.

Kosek, Jake. *Understories: The Political Life of Forests in Northern New Mexico*. Duke University Press, 2006.

Morioka, Rika. "Gender Difference in Risk Perception Following the Fukushima Nuclear Plant Disaster." *Fukushima Global Communication Programme Working Paper Series*, vol. 12, 2015, pp. 1-11.

Morris-Suzuki, Tessa. "Touching the Grass: Science, Uncertainty and Everyday Life from Chernobyl to Fukushima." *Science, Technology & Society*, vol. 19, no. 3, 2014, 331-62.

Paine, Robert. "Danger and the No-Risk Thesis." *Catastrophe & Culture: The Anthropology of Disaster*, edited by Susanna M Hoffman and Anthony Oliver-Smith, School of American Research Press, 2002, pp. 67-89.

Polleri, Maxime. "Tracking Radioactive Contamination after Fukushima." *Anthropology Now*, vol. 8, no. 2, 2016, pp. 90-103.

Sakiyama, Hisako. *Haha to ko no tame no hibaku chishiki—genpatsu jiko kara shokuhin osen made*. Tokyo: Shinsuisha, 2011.

Schrader, Astrid. "Responding to *Pfiesteria Piscicida* (the Fish Killer): Phantomatic Ontologies, Indeterminacy and Responsibility in Toxic Microbiology." *Social Studies of Science*, vol. 40, no. 2, 2010, pp. 275-306.

Slater, David H., et al. "Micro-politics of Radiation: Young Mothers Looking for a Voice in Post-3.11 Fukushima." *Critical Asian Studies*, vol. 46, no. 3, 2014, pp. 485-508.

Sternsdorff-Cisterna, Nicolas. "Food after Fukushima: Risk and Scientific Citizenship in Japan." *American Anthropologist*, vol. 117, no. 3, 2015, pp. 455-67.

Waterton, Claire and Brian Wynne. "Knowledge and Political Order in the European Environment Agency." *States of Knowledge: The Co-production of Science and Social Order*, edited by Sheila Jasanoff, Routledge, 2004, pp. 87-108.

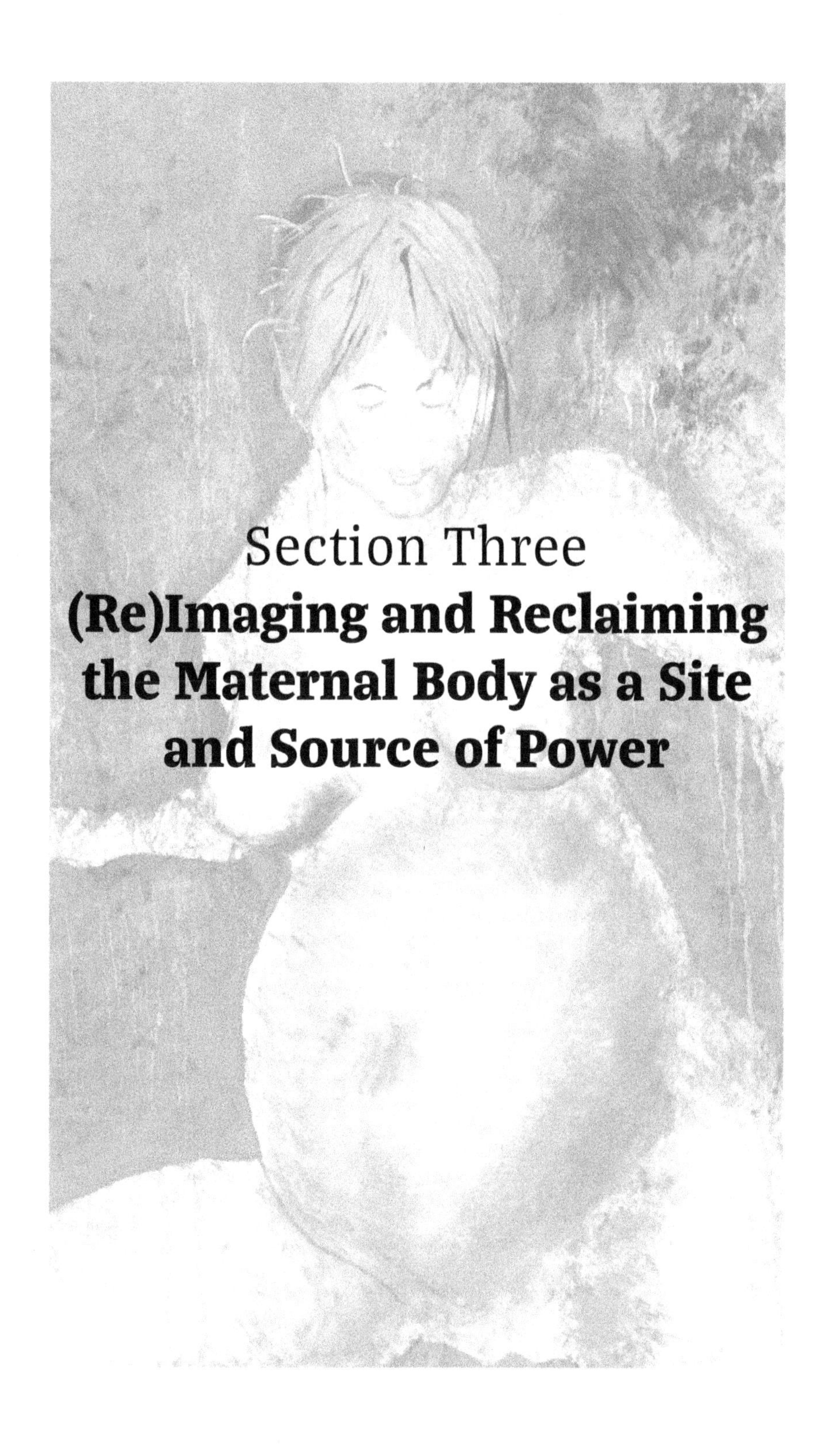

Section Three

(Re)Imaging and Reclaiming the Maternal Body as a Site and Source of Power

Chapter Nine

The Limitations and Possibilities of Genetic Imagery

Jen Rinaldi

Logics of geneticization inform biomedical and social readings of maternal and fetal bodies. Ultrasound imagery has long been held to produce artifacts inextricable from their political interpretation, never simply a one-to-one correspondence with the real. But largely absent from these analyses has been accountings of chromosomal sampling—how they, too, encode the human body to tell a story in relation to genetic normativity and determinism.

In this chapter, I answer the following question: what do chromosomal and chemical renderings of the fetus signify about the maternal body and its relationship to fetal development? Within and through biomedical discourses, prenatal diagnostic strategies such as amniocentesis and chorionic villus sampling are deployed to ideologically organize representations of species-typicality and genetic defect. These prenatal strategies carry sociopolitical force when their interpretations frame bodies as ab/normal at the molecular level in ways that once isolated but now implicate social influence. Against these geneticized logics, I posit alternate accounts of genetics using feminist new materialisms, according to which the agential intra-active properties of the biological work with and through the social. These accounts reveal new possibilities for using prenatal diagnostic technologies and interpreting the genetic readings they produce with more expansive, intercorporeal, and somatechnic frames of analysis, which centre, without responsiblizing, maternal embodiment.

Sights and Signs

Obstetric ultrasound enables the visualization of sound by portraying on a screen the echoes radiating through a uterus, usually against and through liquid (see Figure 1). That this imagery comes to signify anything more than synesthetic effect—anything more than static waves and white noise—requires interpretive and associative work. The inventor of obstetric ultra-sonography, Ian Donald, first interpreted ultrasound imagery through his own system of signification. His intention was to put to rest "the dirty lie that the foetus is just a nondescript meaningless jelly, disposable at will" (qtd. in Nicolson and Fleming 243). From its conception, the image was meant to be imbued with meaning. Feminist scholars have explored how ultrasound has been used to reify the conceptual separation of maternal and fetal bodies, even the displacement of the fetus from the womb (Colker; Katz Rothman; Mitchell). The rendering of the fetus as a distinct entity has implications for the maternal body.

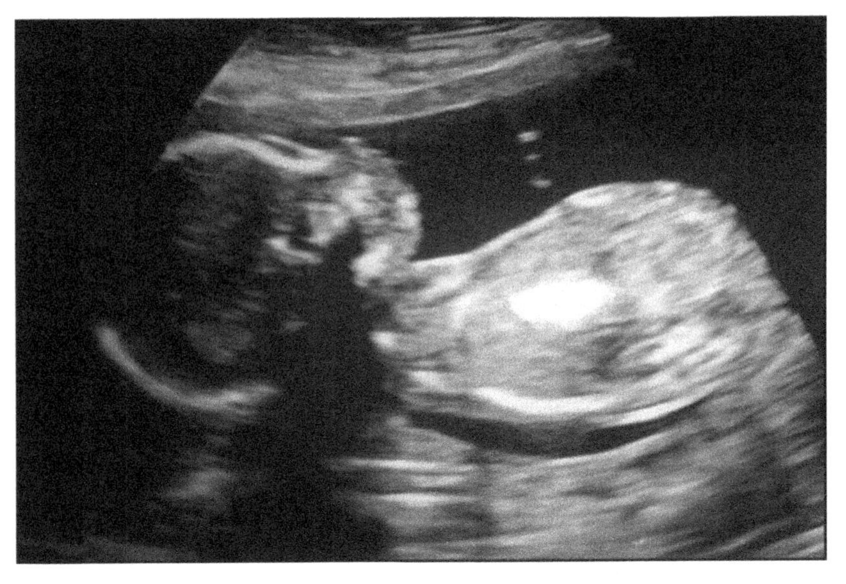

Figure 1. An ultrasound of a fetus in the second trimester of pregnancy. The family photograph is used with the mother's permission.

The writing out of the womb from fetal development is political work that figures into the fetal depictions common to antiabortion campaigns. Put another way: "the technological removal of the fetus from the 'secrecy of the womb' through ultrasound and other prenatal procedures gives the fetus social recognition as an individual separate from the mother" (Blank 73). Feminist political scientist Rosalind P. Petchesky considers how ultrasound imagery has been incorporated into antiabortion campaigns that render "foetal personhood a self-fulfilling prophecy by making the foetus a public presence [in] a visually oriented culture" (263). The fetus of the ultrasound was injected with political signification, and became the posterchild of campaigns opposing abortion, a symbol to rally behind.

It is possible to examine other reproductive technologies in a similar fashion: asking what these technologies are employed to do or what political work they accomplish. Prenatal diagnosis of fetal impairments has extended to tools beyond ultrasonography—which itself is not simply used to determine fetal sex and position, but can now detect gastrointestinal tract anomalies, urinary tract anomalies, congenital heart defects, and skeletal dysplasia—to include invasive prenatal testing procedures. These procedures are available to all pregnant persons in Canada but are especially recommended when pregnancies entail risks of chromosomal anomalies (MacKay and Fraser). Conducted under ultrasonic supervision, amniocentesis procedures extract amniotic fluid between fifteen and seventeen weeks of pregnancy to test for alpha fetoprotein, the concentration of which signals a range of defects. Chorionic villus sampling (CVS) is a transvaginal or trans-abdominal procedure at eleven to twelve weeks of pregnancy, which extracts placental cells to determine the fetus's karyotype profile (Wieacker and Steinhard). Karyotype refers to the characteristics of chromosomal materials, in which anomalies can indicate neural defect (see Figure 2).

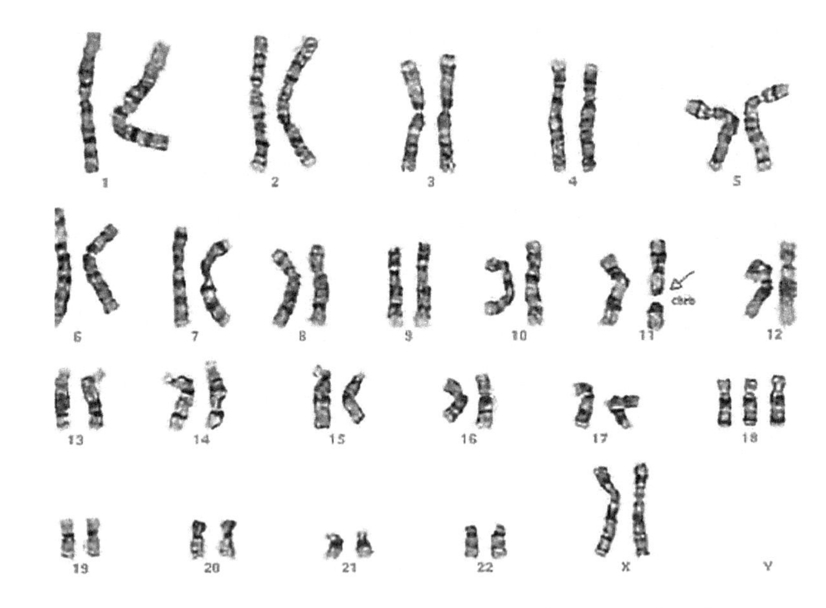

Figure 2. A karyotype profile of a fetus diagnosed with trisomy 18, a chromosomal disorder. The arrow in the eleventh sequence is pointing to a break in the chain, a diagnostic marker (Wieacker and Steinhard).

It may be hard to imagine alpha fetoprotein levels and karyotype analysis are the new ultrasound; matching pairs of lines, like bent segments of worm or friendship bracelets, have so little of the personifying force of ultrasound static, which at least takes a humanoid shape. Yet all these visual products of prenatal diagnosis are studied for their emulation of or variation from a standard portrait. Specifically, chromosomal samples build a karyotype profile for the fetus to which the cells belong, and are compared to the profile befitting a fetus without neural tube defect. The pictures produced mark "the body from which the cells were extracted ... by difference" (Martin 15), particularly in the break in the eleventh sequence in Figure 2.

Visual depictions of genetic materials have come to be interpreted in a fashion comparable to the success of the fetal sonographic image. As Gordon Fyfe and John Law argue in their sociological anthology on visual depiction and social relation, "A depiction is never just an illustration"; it is instead "the material representation, the apparently stabilised product of social difference" (1). Meaning, amniocentesis and CVS use uterine materials to explain and fix what fetal genetics look like, and what they should look like. Rather than trusting the pictures drawn, it is possible instead to "inquire into [a visualization's] provenance, and into the social work that it does ... to decode the hierarchies and differences that it naturalises" (1).

Genetic Coding

What then is being naturalized? Genetic information aids in the construction of what feminist scientist Jackie Leach Scully calls the essentialization and reification of species-typical functioning. We may call this geneticization—a term referring to the reduction of persons to their genetic codes (Lippman; Rapp; Rose). According to bioethicist Rayna Rapp, "geneticization is an historically consonant ideology linking individual attributes and social problems as if they could be effectively reshaped or eliminated only in the realm of biomedicine" (215). She goes on to caution against the attribution of human variation to DNA, which has the effect of "foreground[ing] the biological and background[ing] the social, as if they were separable" (215), as if they could be prioritized. What makes us, *us*, gets crammed into microscopic strands woven into our interiors.

Although feminist analysis of genetic research presented so far has cautioned against bracketing out maternal ecology entirely, genetic determinism in more recent iterations of genetic research risks reintroducing maternal ecology in a specific and problematic role. Epigenetic frames involve the study of modified genetic expression. Whereas the genome remains solidly characterized in scientific circles as inherited and "fixed across the life cycle" (Rutherford 18), the concept of the "epigenome"—the epi bringing in what is outside or around genetic coding—"comprises molecular processes that determine how genes are expressed in specific environmental contexts and which can be permanently modified by early life environmental experience" (18). Chromosomes, or the folding together of gene sequences, are unwound through gene expression; this unwinding may be chemically locked, thus not expressed, in interaction with early environmental exposures. Epigenetics, thus, contains all the trappings of genetic determinism to the extent that genes still write our destiny; only the environmental exposures resulting in locked gene expression can be traced back to what, chemically, makes up the womb (Han; Morgan).

Biological anthropologist Julienne Rutherford describes this process as "genetic complexity," or "alterable, flexible genetic code subject to mechanisms that respond to lived experience" (19). She goes on to explain implications for the maternal-fetal relationship: "the fetus develops in the context of a complex gestational ecology that is informed by proximate maternal physiology"; maternal physiology is created through "an almost limitless range of ... political economic, dietary, familial, and additional factors occurring not only during that pregnancy but over" a life course (19). This reading of chromosomal sampling still flirts with determinism, as the plasticity and perfectibility of the gene expression to which human beings are reduced becomes a maternal responsibility (Valdez). In other words, "the story being told now trades biological and genetic determinism for culturally and socially determined defeat" (Han 75). Such a story carries provenance—that is, it is politicized; whereas ultrasonic imagery displaced the fetus from the womb, genetic imagery implicates the womb in fetal development. In this chapter, I am interested in asking the following: can we use the tools and interpret the findings available to us in the genetic research field to tell a different story? In what follows, I work with feminist new materialisms to centre (without responsiblizing) maternal embodiment in fetal genetic development.

Recoding Genetics

Feminist scientists and critical theorists have grappled with biotechnology and epigenetic messaging, and have explored how to make sense of the maternal role in fetal genetic development. Bioethicist Nikolas Rose says this of the potential of reproductive technologies: "these new technologies, then, do not just seek to cure organize damage or disease, nor to enhance health.... Their key feature is their forward vision" (8). This vision could be so bold as to contribute to "the emergence of a new form of person" (Shildrick 152), one that is "always irreducibly embodied" (155). This new person may also be deeply embedded and enmeshed rather than discrete and distinct. Indeed, Bartha Maria Knoppers, who generally studies genomics and policy, reminds us in her critical analysis of biotechnology that "the human at the level of the species ... while in co-evolution and co-adaptation with nature, is more than the sum total of biological ... components" (9). The fetus's coevolution and co-adaptation works with, alongside, and in the body bearing it. Such an interpretation requires a shift in scientific paradigms—to interpretations of genetic imagery that contend with the realities of genetic science without being reductive.

Prenatal diagnostic technologies carry the potential to reshape body boundaries, eliciting a complex definition of self. Says bioethicist Isabel Karpin: "genetic discourses, indifferent to the surface of the body as a marker of identity, demand a more complex understanding of the self… . What happens, for instance, when genetic discourses reveal that we are all 'leaky,' boundaryless, and transgressive?" (195). The question is a provocative one, as it turns on its head the assembly-line efficiency of decoding genetic coding and expression.

Theorists in the field of somatechnics have worked to reconcile the material and the structural, or, to put it even more crudely, to dissolve the divide between nature and nurture. They do so by braiding "soma" and "techne," or by holding that the body operates in a co-constitutive relationship with discursive and disciplinary forces in the world (Steinbock; Sullivan). They do away with the logic that may otherwise characterize the relationship between body and world—that logic according to which there is a world and a body. Conceptualizing a relationship, a bodyworld, blurring this divide recasts the purposes and potentialities of technologies: "technologies are not something we add to or apply to the body, but rather are the means through which bodies are constituted, positioned and lived" (Pugliese and Giannacopoulos 207). Philosopher Rosi Braidotti calls this relationship "meta(l) morphosis," whereby subjectivity is "shot through with technologically mediated social relations" (*Metamorphosis* 228). By this logic, readings of a karyotype profile have missed not only how technologies have made the picture possible, but how myriad sorts of technologies will introduce possibilities for these strands and sequences.

For Braidotti, biological matter is a "vital, self-organizing, and yet non-naturalistic structure" (*Posthuman* 2), which is self-styled through negotiation. Her analysis complements feminist scientist and new materialist Karen Barad's agential realism, according to which "it is through specific agential intra-actions that the boundaries and the properties of the 'components' of phenomena become determinate and that particular embodied concepts become meaningful" (815). Meaning, matter is agential and carries creative force; it develops or becomes in relation to, within, and through social worlds. Barad is careful to introduce the concept of "intra-action" in contrast with "interaction,"—the latter being loaded with the presumption that things exist prior to their confrontation. For her, biological agency materializes through engagement with social forces. Her agential realism marks a return to materialism, a certain qualified valuing of the potential of our genetic coding, which leaves behind the baggage of determinism by supposing our bodies are not fixed by genetics, but are ever becoming, as our habits and discourses and technes unlock our genetic potentialities.

So as Elizabeth Grosz concretely articulates, activities "help constitute the very biological organization of the subject—the subject's height, weight, coloring, even eye color, are constituted as such by a constitutive interweaving of genetic and environmental factors" (42). Let us return to what this all means for the maternal body. We are from inception relational beings, bound up and enmeshed in an intercorporeal framework that is perhaps the most perfect template for body-becoming theory because fetal development and maternal embodiment exemplify co-constitutive growth—one state does not exist without the other. Across duration, they move along a one-becomes-two trajectory, shifting and adapting to and intra-acting with one another in ways that render their boundary lines fluid and porous, as one is in the other, one flows into the other, and one is made through and by and out of the other.

Therefore, the fetal body cannot be reduced to its chromosomal bits, for fetal becoming makes no sense outside its relation to the pregnant body. Remember that Knoppers tells us the human species is more than the sum of its biological parts; Rapp warns one cannot background and bracket out the social against the biological. They are not wrong. A fetus's environment, their first social world, is not the stage and setting of the play, not the background; it is simultaneously their connected and constituting biology. The womb is both its social world and its agential material. To borrow from Braidotti, pregnancy entails the vital, self-organizing, not-entirely-naturalistic structuring of biological material working toward the point of individuation. Along these lines, feminist and nutritionist Natali Valez argues for feminist frameworks to interpret and, thus, support pregnant persons' experiences and choices, lest "clinical translations of epigenetic theories" (13) render the pregnant body nothing more than an environment: "the politics that undergird the selective translations and applications of epigenetics are situated within a scientific and economic milieu that prioritizes individual responsibility and risk" (14). Such a feminist framing, like the materialist feminist frame advanced in this chapter, still features maternal choice to maternal embodiment, and by extension to fetal development, but in a way that makes meaning rather than distributes responsibility.

Concluding Remarks

I hope this argument is not a throwback to antiabortionist rhetoric of fetal potential, or that it responsibilizes the pregnant person for the activities shaping of fetal biology. Baradian agency is not synonymous with autonomy—that feature of personhood denoting self-governance—but is instead materializing and stabilizing ever-in-relation. Fetal matter comes to matter only in relation to how pregnancy is treated and conducted. The fetus only becomes determinate, or meaningful, in relation to a pregnant person's habitus and choices enacted in and through body. The fetus, that genetic bundle, is indistinguishable, only coming to be distinguished, from the maternal body. This chapter is, then, a ballad dedicated to the creative force of maternal embodiment, to its agential capacity.

This chapter is also an effort to rehabilitate the image of the gene and to reconfigure the role of technology—and its accompanying politics—in pregnancy. Prenatal diagnostic technologies have a habit of narrowing our gaze, and genetically deterministic interpretations of their artifacts have a tendency to presume that selfhood is ready made. Karpin, however, implores us to understand these technologies as the means for dissolving corporeal barriers. They find their way into the womb, digging deep into placental and amniotic fluid, to tell a story about our biology. More than that, they reveal the potential of biology—its animacy in processes of becoming, of individuation and creation, of figuring itself into and being constituted through a biosocial world.

That biosocial world is at the outset the maternal body. The person who chooses their pregnancy and who chooses to usher the fetus into being operates at the threshold of the biological and the social. Maternal embodiment then functions as the fetus's first encounters, first intra-actions, and first conditions for the possibility of becoming. The science of prenatal screening technologies does not unveil complete and intact genetic destinies because absent consideration of the role of pregnancy, it can only glimpse potentiality.

Works Cited

Barad, Karen. "Getting Real: Technoscientific Practices and the Materialization of Reality." *Differences: A Journal of Feminist Cultural Studies*, vol. 10, no. 2, 1998, pp. 87-126.

Blank, Robert H. "Maternal-Fetal Relationship: The Courts and Social Policy." *Journal of Legal Medicine*, vol. 14, 1993, pp. 73-92.

Braidotti, Rosi. *Metamorphosis: Towards a Materialist Theory of Becoming*. Polity Press, 2002.

Braidotti, Rosi. *The Posthuman*. Polity Press, 2013.

Colker, Ruth. *Abortion and Dialogue: Pro-Choice, Pro-Life, and American Law*. Indiana University Press, 1992.

Fyfe, Gordon, and Law, John. *Picturing Power: Visual Depiction and Social Relations*. Routledge, 1988. Grosz, Elizabeth A. *Volatile Bodies: Toward a Corporeal Feminism*. Indiana University Press, 1994.

Han, Sallie. "Pregnant with Ideas: Concepts of the Fetus in the Twenty-First Century United States." *The Anthropology of the Fetus: Biology, Culture, and Society*, edited by Sallie Han et al., Berghahn, 2018, pp. 59-70.

Karpin, Isabel. "Genetics and the Legal Conception of Self." *Ethics of the Body: Postconventional Challenges*, edited by Margrit Shildrick and Roxanne Mykitiuk. The MIT Press, 2005, pp. 195-216.

Katz Rothman, Barbara. *The Tentative Pregnancy: Prenatal Diagnosis and the Future of Motherhood*. Penguin, 1987.

Katz Rothman, Barbara. *Recreating Motherhood: Ideology and Technology in a Patriarchal Society*. Norton, 1999.

Knoppers, Bartha Maria. "Biotechnology: The Human as Biological Resource?" *2006 Killam Annual Lecture*. Trustees of the Killam Trusts, 2006.

Lippman, Abby. "Prenatal Genetic Testing and Geneticization: Mother Matters for All." *Fetal Diagnosis and Therapy*, vol. 8, no. 1, 1993, pp. 175-88.

Martin, Amy. "Genome Presence: The Work of a Diagnostic/Iconic Image." *FES Outstanding Graduate Student Paper Series*, vol. 6, no. 5, 2002.

Mitchell, Lisa M. *Baby's First Picture: Ultrasound and the Politics of the Fetal Subjects.* University of Toronto Press, 2001.

Morgan, Lynn M. *Icons of Life: A Cultural History of Human Embryos.* University of California Press, 2009.

Nicolson, Malcolm, and John EE Fleming. *Imaging and Imagining the Fetus: The Development of Obstetric Ultrasound.* Johns Hopkins University Press, 2013.

Petchesky, Rosalind Pollack. "Fetal Images: The Power of Visual Culture in the Politics of Reproduction." *Feminist Studies*, vol. 13, 1987, pp. 263-92.

Pugliese, Joseph, and Maria Giannacopoulos. "The Lex of Somatechnics." *Griffith Law Review*, vol. 18, no. 2, 2009, pp. 207-11.

Rapp, Rayna. *Testing Women, Testing the Fetus: The Social Impact of Amniocentesis in America.* Routledge, 1999.

Rose, Nikolas. *Politics of Life Itself: Biomedicine, Power and Subjectivity in the Twenty-First Century.* Princeton University Press, 2007.

Rutherford, Julienne. "The Borderless Fetus: Temporal Complexity of the Lived Fetal Experience." *The Anthropology of the Fetus: Biology, Culture, and Society*, edited by Sallie Han, et al., Berghahn, 2018, pp. 15-33.

Scully, Jackie Leach. *Disability Bioethics: Moral Bodies, Moral Difference.* Rowman and Littlefield Publishers, 2008.

Shildrick, Margrit. "Genetics, Normativity, and Ethics: Some Bioethical Concerns." *Feminist Theory*, vol. 5, no. 2, 2004, pp. 149-65."

Steinbock, Bonnie. "Disability, Prenatal Screening, and Selective Abortion." *Prenatal Testing and Disability Rights*, edited by Erik Parens and Adrienne Asch, Georgetown University Press, 2000, pp. 108-23.

Sullivan, Nikki. "The Somatechnics of Perception and the Matter of the Non/Human: A Critical Response to the New Materialism." *European Journal of Women's Studies*, vol. 19, no. 3, 2012, pp. 299-313. P

Valdez, Natali. "The Redistribution of Reproductive Responsibility: On the Epigenetics of 'Environment' in Prenatal Interventions." *Medical Anthropology Quarterly*, 2018, pp. 1-18.

Wieacker, Peter, and Johannes Steinhard. "The Prenatal Diagnosis of Genetic Diseases."*Deutsches Arzteblatt International*, vol. 107, no. 48, 2010, pp. 857-62.

Chapter Ten

Feeding the World: Reconsidering the Multibreasted Body of Artemis Ephesia

Carla Ionescu

Tabooed, worshipped, and sometimes exploited, the female breast is a visible, tangible, and beautiful feature of the female body. Although the female breast is a secondary sexual organ and is not necessary for reproduction, it has an aesthetic and a functionality making it distinctly female. The breast is physiologically a mammary gland designed to provide nourishment to newborn babies, yet its physical feature, its sensitivity, and its oral practicality have created a fascination influencing the value placed on it both by men and women (Jones 15).

To understand contemporary attitudes about the female breast, it is necessary to analyze traditional and persistent symbolism and imagery around the concept of breastfeeding as providing natural substance that has influenced modern Western culture. In monotheistic cultures such as Judaism, Christianity, and Islam, the breast manifested sacredness and was believed to be the "spiritual nurturance of all Christian souls" (Yalom 5). This tradition harkens back to the Paleolithic period (approx. 10,000 BCE), as archaeologists have found female figurines from this period sculpted out of bone, stone, or clay, with prominent breasts, and a voluptuous female figure believed to be a symbolism of fertility and healthy offspring. This chapter will examine the primordial, exhilarating, and monstrous image of the multibreasted goddess Artemis Ephesia through the overlapping influence of art and sculpture as well as the discourse of mothering roles and identities reflected in Mother Goddess ritual and tradition.

Ancient Mother Goddesses

In examining the origins of the concept of Mother Goddess, scholars are presented with a massive collection of archaeological and anthropological data representing both folk and popular practices as well as cultic ritual and religious tradition. The Neolithic age of human development beginning in the ancient Eastern Mediterranean around 8500 BCE, and gradually reaching the northern tip of Scotland by 3000 BCE, has left archaeology with little documented evidence other than cult objects and cult places (Holladay 268-69). Many of these objects are female figurines often carved out of bone or stone depicting larger-than-life female bodies with ample breasts and hips.

One of the most worshiped deities of the ancient world was the Phrygian goddess Cybele. This deity may have evolved from an Anatolian Mother Goddess whose ritual remnants might have been found at Çatalhöyük and date back to the sixth-millennium BCE. Walter Burkert places her among the "foreign gods" of Greek religion—a complex figure combining the Minoan-Mycenaean tradition with the Phrygian cult imported directly from Asia Minor (177). One of the earliest material depictions of the "Great Mother" is described by Sarolta Takács as a terracotta statuette of a seated (mother) goddess giving birth with each hand on the head of a leopard or panther (376). In Phrygian art of the eighth-century BCE, the cult attributes of the Phrygian Mother Goddess include attendant lions, a bird of prey, and a small vase for her libations or other offerings (Simpson 198-201).

In the second-century CE, Pausanias attested to a Magnesian (Lydian) cult to "the Mother of the Gods" whose image was carved into a rock spur of Mount Sipylus. During this period, it was believed to be the oldest image of the goddess, and was attributed to the legendary Broteas. As Pausanias writes: "the Magnesians, who live to the north of Spil Mount, have on the rock Coddinus the most ancient of all the images of the Mother of the gods. The Magnesians say that it was made by Broteas the son of Tantalus" (3.22.4). The gigantic remains of such a figure at Mount Sipylus, though lacking inscriptions and much eroded, are consistent with later representations of a seated Cybele, with a supporting or attendant lion beneath each arm. At Pessinos in Phrygia, the Mother Goddess, as identified by Pausanias as Cybele, took the form of an unshaped stone of black meteoric iron, and might have been associated with, or identical to, Agdistis, Pessinos's mountain deity. In his description of the story of Cybele/Agdistis's birth, Pausanias translates the names of the Phrygian sky god into Greek as Zeus and the earth goddess as Gaia: "Zeus [or rather the Phrygian sky god], it is said, let fall in his sleep seed upon the ground, which in course of time sent up a Daimon, with two sexual organs, male and female. They call the Daimon Agdistis [Cybele]. But the gods, fearing Agdistis, cut off the male organ" (Pausanias 7.17.8). No contemporary text or myth survives to attest the original character and nature of Cybele's Phrygian cult. Images and iconography in funerary contexts, and the ubiquity of her Phrygian name "Matar" or Mother, suggest she was a mediator between the "boundaries of the known and unknown" (Roller 110-14): the civilized and the wild, the worlds of the living and the dead

From around the sixth-century BCE, cults to the Anatolian Mother Goddess were introduced from Phrygia into the ethnically Greek colonies of Western Anatolia, mainland Greece, the Aegean islands and the westerly colonies of Magna Graecia. The Greeks called her "*Mātēr*" or "*Mētēr* Mother," or from the early fifth century, *Kubelē*. The great Greek poet Pindar (522 - 443 BCE) refers to her as Mistress Cybele the Mother (Roller 125). In Greece, as in Phrygia, she was *Potnia Therōn* or Queen of Beasts[1]; her mastery of the natural world was expressed by the lions flanking her, sitting on her lap or drawing her chariot. She was readily assimilated to the Minoan-Greek earth-mother Rhea, "Mother of the Gods," whose raucous, ecstatic rites she might have acquired. As an exemplar of devoted motherhood, she was partly assimilated to the grain-goddess Demeter, whose torchlight procession recalled her search for her lost daughter, Persephone (Roller 170-76).

It is easy to understand how the attributes of Cybele were easily incorporated into the characteristics of the Greek Artemis. There are significant overlapping similarities making Artemis the best possible heir to these ancient traditions. Arriving with the Greeks, Artemis the Huntress is already mistress of the animals, and in this form, she is flanked by a variety of wild beasts. As the goddess of childbirth and the divinity of transitions, she is in the best position to take over all the nurturing, life-giving responsibilities. The one aspect Artemis Ephesia strictly inherits from Cybele and her Anatolian roots is the position as Mother Goddess or the Great Mother. If Pausanias is correct in his retelling of the legend in which Agdistis (Zeus) removes his male genitals and becomes a female goddess Cybele, then one can argue that Cybele/Artemis embodies both male and female qualities and is, therefore, a complete parthenogenetic[2] divinity.This explains why Artemis Ephesia is constantly referred to as queen and reigns supreme in the Ephesus pantheon.

Frederick Brenk argues this dual iconography indicates the double nature of Artemis Ephesia as a co-opted Anatolian goddess reenvisioned as the Greek Artemis; the inclusion of the "Ephesia" type of the goddess was an effort by Ephesus to portray the unique Anatolian provenance of their Artemis to the greater Roman world (Brenk 160). Hans Willer Laale supports this claim and suggests that for the sake of unity, the population of Ephesus gradually commingled its religious beliefs and practices. By doing so, they changed the revered image of the Greek Artemis of the Hunt, the twin sister of Apollo, into the many-breasted statue of Artemis Ephesia, which embodies the native Anatolian Mother Goddess Cybele (Laale 9).

Artemis Ephesia: The Multibreasted Body

When early Christians first saw the multibreasted Artemis Ephesia, located in her Temple at Ephesus, they were appalled by the monstrosity of her mammalian body. As worshipers of an incarnate male god, they struggled with the complexity of a multibreasted body, a body that feeds the entire world.

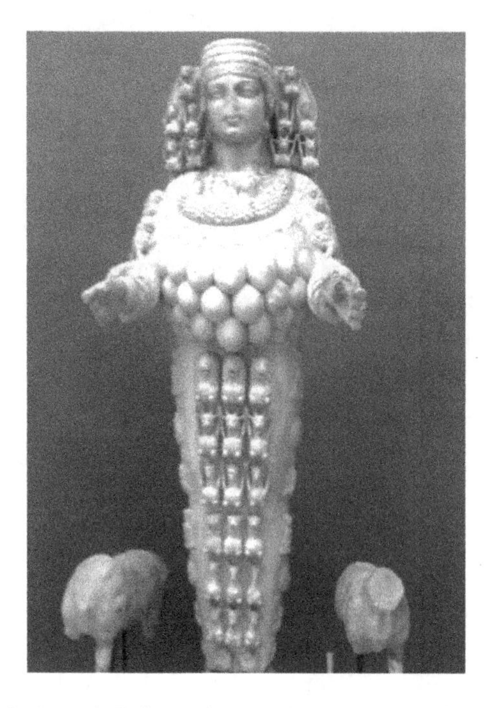

Figure 1. Artemis Ephesia, National Archaeological Museum, Naples, Italy

Artemis is a goddess of totality. In many aspects she is the Saviour *Sôteira*, the Light Bringer *Phosphorus*, the One Who Soothes, *Hêmerasia*. In others, she is Huntress of the Wilds, *Agrotera*, who delights in the Showering of Arrows, *Iokheaira*, she who rigorously protects her chastity, which is reflected in her titles as Virgin or Maiden *Parthenos*, as well as Revered Virgin *Aedoeus Parthenos*. Most importantly, she is a Royal Princess, *Basileis*, a goddess Of the First Throne, *Protothronia*, who reigns unmatched throughout the Mediterranean as Goddess Queen, *Potnia Thea* (Redfield 129). This multitude of titles, attributes, incarnations, and constant adaptation provide more than sufficient evidence that Artemis is the Goddess for all peoples at all times in all places. Her cult worship is as varied as the people who devote themselves to her. This diversity reflects the goddess's sphere of influence as both the agent through which community history is inherited as well as the medium through which community culture is maintained. Her devotees are not a uniform cult simply transported from one place to another, from one time to another, but an array of various forms of worship embedded within each locality and its unique cultural practices all under the aegis of Artemis.

One of the most significant differences between the Artemis of Ephesus and the Greek Artemis can be found in the foundational myths of her Anatolian heritage. Whereas the Greek Artemis embodies many aspects of nature, rites of passage, and involvement in the life of her followers, the Artemis of Ephesus represents a much more complicated and powerful divinity. Artemis Ephesia originates from the Mother of the Gods herself. Her direct connection through the Amazons to the goddess Cybele places her in a position of power—the likes of which the Greek Artemis could never reach. The ancient Greek depicted the Amazons as a nation of warrior women, and numerous stories describe how these women would chop off their right breast to strengthen their right arm and facilitate the drawing of the bow (Yalom 22). Greek myth depicts numerous heroes and demigods such as Heracles and Perseus who battle the Amazons as equals in strength, athleticism, and self-sacrifice. The myth of these warrior women describes them abandoning their male children and keeping only their female offspring as new recruits. There is an evident connection here between the lack of breasts and lack of mothering. The Amazons are not portrayed as nurturing mothers, primarily because they are physically incapable of nurturing their infants.

There are two aspects of Artemis Ephesia presenting her as foundationally different from her Greek counterpart. First, she was established in the area of Ephesus as a powerful deity. Legends say the Amazons created her powerful preeminence. (Farnell 481). This connection explains in part the fearsome and authoritative position Artemis holds in Ephesus. Here, she is not merely the goddess of the Hunt; she is a warrior goddess, a mother, a creator, and the powerful source of the embodiment of divine strength. Whether or not they existed—the ancient Greeks thought they did—the Amazons were not only feared but also respected. This respect was not due to their representation as women, but to their mythological skill as soldiers. Thus, since the Amazons were viewed as tribal women who were unbending, nonconforming, and unforgiving, their goddess had to be equally unrelenting and severe.

The second aspect making Artemis Ephesia different from her Greek counterpart is her Cretan inheritance. The Greek Artemis incorporated some early Minoan and Mycenaean characteristics. Most of these involved being the Mistress of Animals, a nature goddess, and a nurturing divinity. And although these provide the Greek Artemis with a significant amount of influence, her main identity remains as an Olympian daughter, sister, and helper. In contrast, the Artemis of Ephesus inherits the characteristics, responsibilities, and authority, of the Cretan "Mother of Gods"—Cybele (Farnell 379). This inheritance provides Artemis Ephesia with a powerful royal lineage, a worldly responsibility, and a complete dominion over all Ephesian citizens. The "Mother of Gods" attribute is a foundational difference transforming the traditional Greek attributes of Artemis into a whole new dimension: she rivals the authority and influence of Zeus. Thus, in Ephesus, Artemis is not just an Olympian. As Cybele, her authority predates the Olympians, and through this early Cretan practice, she embodies the Titan Rhea, and even the all-encompassing Mother Goddess Gaia (Nilsson 211).

Apart from her name, it would be difficult to recognize the Greek Artemis in the deity of Ephesus. The sacred statue of Artemis Ephesia is described as an image attired in a "*polymastros,*" or a multibreasted vest, wearing a turret crown on her head. The turret-crown, later to be a significant feature on the head of the cult statue, symbolizes that she, like Cybele, oversees the wellbeing of her people (Farnell 481). Traditionally, scholars have interpreted her breasts as perhaps representing eggs, acorns, scrotum of bulls, bags of amulets, or other elements. Patrick Clayton explains the following: "The peculiar many breasted statue of Artemis Ephesia represents a Mother Goddess, the breast symbolizing the fertility of women. The statue is rigid, the lower portion like an Egyptian mummy case. The decorative elements, stags, bulls, lions, griffins, sphinxes, sirens, these, are creatures originally of the East" (87). This image was made out of wood, set upright, and fastened so that it would not topple. According to Pausanias, it was an image of "a goddess held in honour above all else" (4 31.8). Callimachus recites how the Amazons would dance around the sacred sculpture in preparation for their battles.

In addition to the shared characteristics between Artemis and the Mistress of Animals, Nilsson further suggests that the worship of Artemis also contains remnants of an equally popular Minoan divinity, the goddess of Nature. The Minoan Nature goddess was a goddess of fertility, not of agrarian fertility, but of the fertility of humans and animals. She assisted women in the pangs of childbirth; she fostered young animals and the small children of man. She is intimately connected with one form of the tree cult, established around the sacred Bo tree, which conveys life and fertility (Nilsson 389). Artemis inherits such characteristics; she is a goddess of fertility, particularly in her Ephesian incarnation, she helps women in childbirth and she is often worshiped in the guise of a tree. Pausanias describes her worship as a myrtle tree in Boiai, a village in Lakedaimonia, as follows "they built a city on the site of the myrtle, and down to this day they worship that myrtle tree, and name Artemis *Sôteira* [Saviour]" (Pausanias 3.22.12). Martin Nilsson notes that there is a close connection between the goddess of the tree cult and the Mistress of Animals. Both being nature goddesses, it would not be unnatural to regard them as forms of the same deity (Price 399). Consequently, Artemis inherits the attributes of the Mistress of Animals, whose close associations with other Minoan goddesses of nature would also be inherited. Again, she embodies the imagery, weapons, responsibilities, and attributes of her earlier counterparts, which provides further evidence that Artemis is not a divinity created by the Greeks as part of their pantheon, but a goddess that was already deeply rooted in Mycenaean territory, who was more easily transfigured into a goddess that could be categorized as Greek than removed.

Some of the well-known titles for Artemis are related to nature, such as goddess of the hunt, the lake, the oak tree. However, many of her other titles are closely related to her role in the salvation and mercy she granted her followers. Such names include the following: *Orsilochia* or Helper of Childbirth; *Selasphoros and/or Phôsphoros* or Light-Bringer; *Hêmerasia* or She who Soothes; and *Hymniê* Of the Hymns. These names proclaim Artemis's significance in the lives of her followers both as healer, and as a mother figure. Consequently, this suggests that Artemis was in fact "the People's Goddess," and that her followers relied on her mercy to get through the gruelling tasks of living.

Before the Virgin Mary was given authority over the domain of nurturing and protecting her followers, the Greek Artemis was worshiped under several titles of caregiver and protector. While at Ephesus, Artemis Ephesia was expressively viewed as a goddess of fertility and protection. Some of the titles of worship for Artemis include the following: *Philomeirax*, Friend of Young Girls; *Paidotrophos*, Nurse of Children; *Orsilokhia*, Helper of Childbirth; and *Hêmerasia*, She who Soothes (Callimachus 3.21-2). The epithets served as foundations on which the people of Ephesus could adapt Artemis into the realm of Kybele, *Magna Mater*—the Mother Goddess who ruled this area from archaic times and through the early Hellenistic period.

At the core of the worship of Artemis Ephesia was the belief in her position as fertility goddess and mother to her people. Scholars often discuss her association with childbirth and her role as protector of the young. In Callimachus's *Hymn to Artemis*, Artemis declares that because her own mother gave birth to her without pain, she will be forever the protector of pregnant women, or women in childbirth (3.21-2). She is also revered as the saviour of all women—particularly those who have been unfairly treated by men—but she also presides over wedding feats, assists women in becoming pregnant, and watches over the offspring of her followers. According to Dieter Knibbe, the Ephesians had been performing animal sacrifices as fertility rites in her temple for hundreds of years:

> There were offerings of incense and according to the bones found in the Artemision sacrifices of a great variety of animals. On certain occasions a series of bulls were offered to the goddess in bloody slaughter and it was suggested by early Swiss archaeologists that their testicles were fixed on the statue of Artemis this right reveals the archaic concept that the power of the goddess was renewed in this way so that she could intern strengths in the world of nature and allow even the dead to receive a share of her vitality (142).

Thus, Artemis was not only the mistress of earth fertility, but also the protector of the dead. Knibbe states that she visited the dead from time to time in a procession on her sacred way around Mount Pion (Knibbe 142). The sacred way was originally a cemetery encircling the entire mountain. Consequently, Artemis inherits all fertility rituals; she takes on the responsibilities of life and death, and of nourishment and protection, which originally belonged to the Phrygian Mother.

Artemis Ephesia's most notable responsibility is her role as guardian of the inhabitants of Ephesus. The turret crown she wears in Ephesus symbolizes that she, like Cybele, oversees the wellbeing of her people

(Farnell 481). According to Rachel Lesser, the Ephesians are often called the "nurslings" of their goddess (Lesser 46). In addition, Callimachus refers to her as "Upis Queen" (237-58) in his discussion of the founding of the Ephesian cult in his *Hymn to Artemis*. Farnell notes that the title "*Upis*" was a name of Artemis that the Greeks interpreted as "watcher" (488).

At Ephesus, Artemis Ephesia was famously known as the many-breasted Mother Goddess, a tradition that traces back to the Anatolian Kybele. Traditionally, scholars have discussed the polymastoid (mammarylike) nature of the top body of her statue as representative of breasts, the scrotums of bulls, eggs, acorns, or bags of amulets. Clayton states that the globelike protrusions must be breasts, as they are a definitive symbol of the Mother Goddess: "The peculiar many breasted statue of Artemis Ephesian represents a Mother Goddess, the breasts symbolizing the fertility of women" (87). Whether the statue of Artemis Ephesia wears many breasts, bull scrota, or beehives, she represents nourishment and fertility; she is the benefactor of her people who bestows on them the sacred gift of milk and honey. As with the Virgin Mary, she allows her followers to feed from her body, and her icons represent the connections between the natural fertility of Mother Goddess and the health, wellbeing, and sustenance of her people.

Suckling and Lactation: The Breast that Feeds the World

Goddesses suckling their divine offspring can be traced back to the earliest civilizations. Two thousand years before Christ, the goddess of Ur offered her son her breasts; a thousand years later, in Egypt, Isis nourishes Horus; in Mexico, statues dated to 1000 BCE have been discovered of female deities nursing their babies (Feininger and Bon 38). On the African continent, along the Lower Congo, the Ivory Coast, and the Gold Coast, sacred mothers nurse their sacred infants, and in India, sculptures show the infant Krishna with his mother Devaki (41). This natural nourishment and bond of mother to child has been celebrated, honoured, and ritualized by human beings as far back as history is traced. Thus, it is not surprising to find the image of the Virgin Mary nursing Jesus in early Christian literature and art. Although the Virgin as mother was exempt from intercourse or labour in Christianity, she was permitted to suckle (Warner 192). Marina

Warner states the following: "Milk symbolized the full humanity of Jesus at one level, but it also belonged in an ancient and complex symbolic language. For milk was a crucial metaphor of the gift of life.... The milk of the Mother of God became even more highly charged with the symbolism of life, for the life of life's own source depended on it" (192).

Consequently, Mary's milk can nourish and feed the divine in Jesus, which becomes intertwined with the Christian mystery of the incarnate God. This is no ordinary mother feeding her child; this is not even a goddess mother feeding a goddess son. This is a human woman, albeit a special human woman, suckling the divine, whose human body nourishes the man who is the vehicle for humanity's salvation. In the apocryphal *Odes of Solomon*, written before the third century, milk is the agent of conception of the *logos* (or the word of God). Mary describes the virgin birth as a series of exchanges of wisdom and power: "A cup of milk was offered to me: and I drank it in the sweetness of the delight of the Lord. The son is the cup, and He who is milked is the Father, and the Holy Spirit milked Him, because his breasts were full, and it was necessary for him that his milk should be sufficiently released" (Boslooper qtd. in Harris 62). Here, milk has a metaphysical significance, which harkens back to classical Greek myth, particularly the upbringing of Zeus, and even Dionysus. As an infant, Zeus was suckled by Amaltheia, who was the wife of Melisseus. Melisseus comes from the word "*melissa*," which can be translated as "bee man." Whereas Amaltheia provided Zeus with milk, her husband provided him with honey. Similarly, in some accounts of the infancy of Dionysus, the nymph Macris raised him on milk and honey (Elderkin et al. 205). Moreover, the physical quality of mother's milk carried the symbolism of purity; white, gleaming, and moist, it was the imagery equivalent to astral light. For the Romans, this connection between milk and the eternity of the heavens is exemplified in the myth of the creation of the Milky Way. Legend claims that one night while nursing Hercules, Juno's milk sprayed across the sky and created the Milky Way, and our galaxy (Elderkin et al. 205). In fact, the Greek word for milk is "*galaktos*."

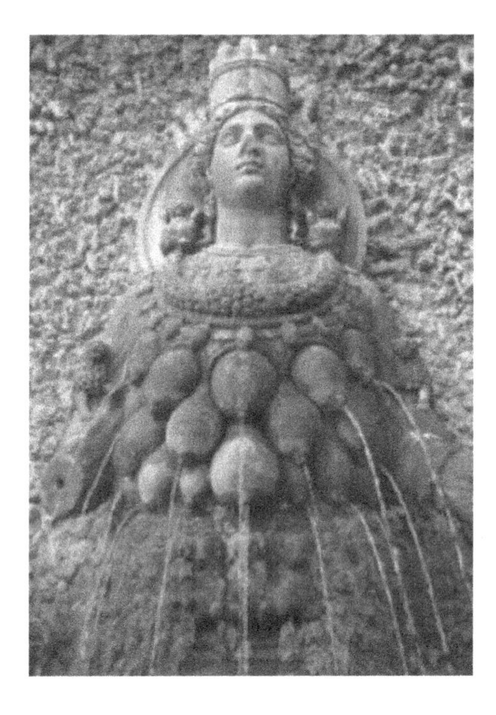

Figure 2. Fountain of Fertility, Diana Efesina, 1569, Villa d'Este, Tivoli

This fascination with lactation and "sacred" milk inspired numerous European artists. Lactating nereids, sirens, and goddesses were, in fact, a manifestation of the high Mannerist style, popular in Italy in the sixteenth century. This visual tradition of representing nature as a lactating woman, or a multibreasted woman, remained in the imagination of Christian converts and became popular symbols for protection, regeneration, and fertility. The *Fountain of Diana Efesina* from 1569, for example, is clear evidence that despite Christianity's continued desiccation of Greco-Roman symbols of worship, the multibreasted goddess—her sacred milk overflowing, her nurturing body sustaining all the world—outlasted all attempts to destroy and forget a polytheistic past.

Multibreasted Natura: Artistic Interpretations of Nature

By the early 1500s, artists recycled and recreated the physical representations of nature, but her polymasterous depiction remained unchanged. In 1528, Niccolo Tribolo sculpted his now famous marble statue *Nature.* This multibreasted representation of the goddess decorates the room of Madame d'Etampes at Fountainbleau, and is an extravagant variation of Artemis Ephesia—her body also covered in animals, birds, and fantastical vegetation (Balas 132). This early style of recreating the goddess speaks to the continued obsession and idealization of the female body, which is at once an embodiment of abundance. and a grotesque or unnatural image of sexuality and pleasure.

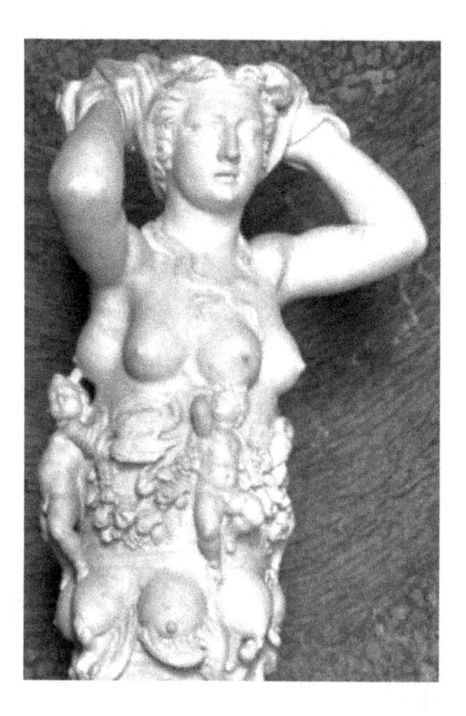

Figure 3. Niccolo Tribolo, Nature, 1528, Madame d'Etampes, Fountableau, France

One hundred years later, in 1681, a similar form of the multibreasted Artemis appeared as a frontispiece for Gerardus Blasius's *Anatome Animalium.* Although Blasius was a practising physician in Amsterdam, his real interest was anatomy, particularly comparative anatomy. He worked closely with philosophers and scientists—such as John Locke, Jan Swammerdam, and Niels Stensen—to promote the study of anatomy and to widen the availability of both animal and human remains for closer study (Tevebring 156). Blasius is a man of science, whose work often emphasizes the importance of intelligence of the human mind as tools to be used to unveil and uncover nature's mysteries. During the sixteenth century, an oppositional battle ensued between the philosophical "thinking" mind and the natural "organic" body. Blasius's frontispiece depicts the female personification of knowledge or science, and unveils the mammary, mysterious, yet no less powerful goddess Natura. According to Frederika Tevebring, "veiled nature in the work of Blasius and Leeuwenhooek is to be understood as literal. Writing on anatomy and the microscope respectively, the two scientists unveiled nature's secrets by opening her up and looking inside her" (157).

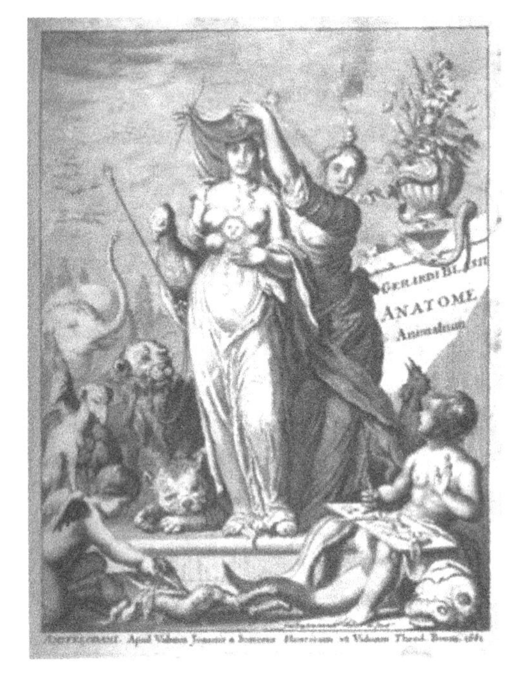

Figure 4. Gerardus Biasius's Anatome Animalium, Amsterdam, 1681

By the late eighteenth century, the multibreasted goddess became a source of disdain and fear. Joseph Anton Koch's *The Painter as Hercules at the Crossroads*, from 1791 (the drawing is now lost), recalls the iconographical convention of showing a hero at a junction where he can choose the direction of either vice or virtue, which is symbolized by two different female figures. The statuesque figure on the left represents art-as-virtue, whereas the other figure, decked out in garish clothing, is "art-as-whore," who binds Koch with a chain around his ankle. The sacred, fascinating symbolism that has uniquely identified Artemis Ephesia as Mother Goddess for thousands of years has become this grotesque figure, both tempting and mocking intellectuals and artists of the Enlightenment.

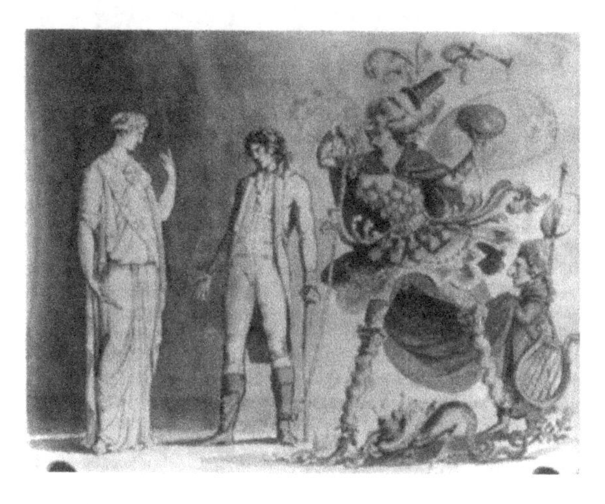

Figure 5. Joseph Anton Koch, The Painter as Hercules at the Crossroads, 1791, Lost drawing

Conclusion

Although the popularity of Artemis Ephesia and her multibreasted representations might have weaned in popularity for the last hundred years, artists are once again revamping her extraordinary body and placing her in central public locations for people to admire and gawk at. In 1993, a large sculpture *Cybele, Goddess of Fertility* by Mihail Chemiakin stood outside the Mimi Ferzt Gallery in New York City, and displayed her abundance for all to see. Was this rendition iconic? Or was it an example of exaggeration and monstrosity in modern imagination? Were tourists and art enthusiasts in awe of her mammalian body, or did they find her grotesque and unnatural?

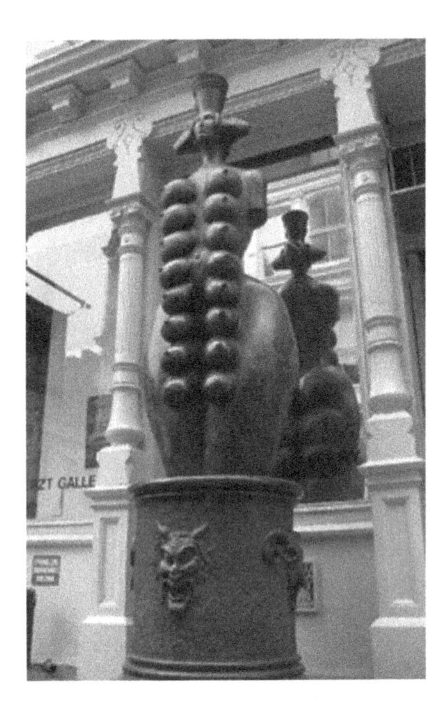

Figure 6. Cybele, Goddess of Fertility, Mikhail Chemiakin,
Mimi Ferzt Gallery, NYC, 1993

There is much still to be uncovered in the study of Mother Goddess worship, particularly in the analysis of the female body as a source of maternal nourishment. Though scholars have combed through archeological data for the last hundred years, Johanna Stuckey argues that the focus on the maternal has been primarily established within a patriarchal framework, and Mother Goddesses have often been overlooked based on their bodily depictions in art and sculpture (33). Consequently, it is no small feat to reclaim and reveal the multifaceted responsibilities, political power, and spiritual influence that the multibreasted goddess had over her worshippers, community, and society. Future research projects should aim to present the role of Artemis Ephesia unilaterally to better understand the relationship between our ancestors and this mighty goddess, and why the symbol of her mammalian figure remains entrenched in our modern imagination.

Endnotes

1 *Potnia Theron* can sometimes be found as a title in ancient sources, but it is also a scholarly inference drawn from iconography (Roller 135).

2 Parthenogenesis can be defined as a type of asexual reproduction in which the offspring develops from unfertilized eggs. In this case, it refers to the ability of some female deities to create offspring without male assistance.

Works Cited

Balas, Edith. *The Mother Goddess in Italian Renaissance Art.* Carnegie Mellon University Press, 2002.

Boslooper, Thomas. *The Virgin Birth.* The Preacher's Library, 1962.

Brenk, Frederick E. *Relighting the Souls: Studies in Plutarch, in Greek Literature, Religion, and Philosophy, and in the New Testament Background.* Franz Steiner Verlag, 1998.

Burkert, Walter. *Greek Religion.* Harvard University Press, 1985.

Callimachus. *Callimachus' Hymns.* Edited by Robert Schmiel, Bryn Mawr College, 1984 Elderkin, George W, et al. *Antioch On-the-Orontes.* Princeton University Press, 1934.

Farnell, Lewis Richard. *Greek Hero Cults and Ideas of Immortality: The Gifford Lectures Delivered in the University of St. Andrews in the Year 1920.* Clarendon, 1921.

Feininger, Andreas, and J Bon. *The Image of Woman: Women in Sculpture from Pre-historic Times to the Present Day.* Thames and Hudson, 1960.

Harris, J Rendell. *Odes and Psalms of Solomon,* Cambridge: The University Press,1909.

Jones, Diana P. "Cultural Views of the Female Breast." *The Association of Black Nursing Faculty Journal,* vol. 15, no. 1, 2004, pp. 15-21.

Knibbe, Dieter. "Via Sacra Ephesiaca: New Aspects of the Cult of Artemis Ephesia." *Ephesos: Metropolis of Asia,* edited by Helmut Koester. Trinity Press International, 1995, pp. 144-73.

Laale, Hans Willer. *Ephesus (Ephesos): An Abbreviated History from Androclus to Constantine XI.* WestBow, 2011.

Lesser, Rachel. "The Nature of Artemis Ephesia." *Hirundo: The McGill Journal of Classical Studies,* vol. 4, 2005-6, pp. 43-54.

Nilsson, Martin P. *The Minoan-Mycenaean Religion and Its Survival in Greek Religion*. Biblo and Tannen, 1971.

Pausanias. *Description of Greece*. Translated by WHS Jones and HA Omerod. Loeb Classical Library Volumes. Harvard University Press, 1918.

Price, M. *The Seven Wonders of the Ancient World*. Routledge, 1996.

Redfield, J. *From Sex to Politics: The Rites of Artemis Triklaria and Dionysus Aisymnētēs at Patras. Before Sexuality*. Princeton University Press. 1990.

Roller, Lynn E. *In Search of God the Mother: The Cult of Anatolian Cybele*. University of California, 1999.

Simpson, Elizabeth. "Phrygian Furniture from Gordion." *The Furniture Of Ancient Western Asia*, edited by Georgina Herrmann, 1996, pp. 198-201.

Stuckey, Johanna. "Ancient Mother Goddesses and Fertility Cults." *Journal of the Association for Research on Mothering*, vol. 7, no. 1, 2005, pp. 32-44.

Warner, M. *Alone of All Her Sex: The Myth and the Cult of the Virgin Mary*. Picador. 1985.

Yalom M. *A History of Breasts*. Alfred A Knopf, 1997.

Chapter Eleven

"I'm MY Breastfeeding Expert": How First-Time Mothers Reclaimed their Power through Breastfeeding

Catherine Ma

Although biomedicine has led to scientific advances in maternal health, its influences on the breastfeeding experiences of mothers have been less positive, often encouraging women to view breastfeeding as an activity relying heavily on the expertise of policymakers and medical professionals. Current views of breastfeeding in the United States are often shaped by government agencies such as the American Academy of Pediatrics and Centers for Disease Control. These agencies play a pivotal role with their breastfeeding guidelines and health promotion strategies—such as the Healthy People 2020 campaign, which aims to have 81.9 percent of all mothers to initiate breastfeeding, 60.6 percent to continue for six months, and 34.1 percent to continue for one year (Eidelman et al. e827; "Breastfeeding Report Card" 2; "Healthy People 2020"). Although many of these agencies acknowledge factors that may reduce breastfeeding rates, their approaches encourage a portrayal of breastfeeding that ignores the complexities inherent in how women learn and experience breastfeeding. Medical professionals often overlook and ignore how a healthy newborn is able to make their way up to their mother's breast and suckle; indeed, hospital procedures that focus on taking babies to the nursery to be cleaned and weighed interrupt this important time between mother and infant (Palmer 20). Ensuing effects of this biomedical influence are healthcare initiatives perpetuating the notion that low rates of breastfeeding are due to a lack of education regarding its health benefits, when in reality, the situation is much more convoluted (Kukla 161). Under this discourse, medical experts and health organizations play a dominant role in shaping how women learn about breastfeeding, which often neglects the voices of the women who perform this important work. Breastfeeding rhetoric internalized by both medical staff and new mothers can instil doubt into the minds of nursing women and encourage a reliance on biomedical practices often leaving out the embodied experiences of the nursing dyad (Tomori 39).

What has been underexplored is the impact of this biomedical model on the lived experiences of first-time mothers learning how to breastfeed. One hundred and twenty first time mothers were followed from their last trimester of pregnancy until the late postpartum period to explore the influence of the biomedical model on their breastfeeding experiences. Although their breastfeeding journeys revealed numerous challenges stemming from following suggestions inherent in the current breastfeeding model, there were also significant triumphs that fostered maternal transformations, as mothers grew empowered from listening to their infants and satisfying their own needs. This chapter reveals how breastfeeding can act as a catalyst toward a deeper understanding of maternal embodiment, in which alternative views of breastfeeding can broaden current conceptions of infant feeding. Through maternal embodiment, breastfeeding becomes a lens in how nursing women can experience motherhood as both idiosyncratic and universal. Imagine if new mothers learned to view breastfeeding as a dynamic process that could teach them to be more confident, empowered, and critical of breastfeeding rules, thus challenging the biomedical model. Sharing the experiences of this group of first-time mothers attempts to make visible the challenges many new mothers face when breastfeeding does not go as expected. By focusing on the lived experiences of these marginalized mothers, breastfeeding researchers and advocates can highlight how adversity can give birth to strength, empowerment, and confidence. These stories of resilience can help other mothers see the light at the end of their often stressful and discouraging journey into breastfeeding.

Biomedical Influence

Whereas a large percentage of research on breastfeeding identifies barriers women face, this chapter focuses on maternal transformations or what women learned about themselves while nursing their newborns. The majority of the women in the sample faced obstacles in their journey into first-time motherhood and breastfeeding, which is not unusual for new mothers. The stories of resilience, humility and resistance from mothers who struggle with breastfeeding, however, are less common. A closer examination of the current breastfeeding paradigm reveals its hidden agendas, which often create impediments hindering women from success. The biomedical influence during the eighteenth century—when pregnancy and breastfeeding came under the rule and control of men in the obstetric profession—has heavily shaped the history of breastfeeding (Palmer 24). Breastfeeding became controlled by medical experts, who often neglected the interdependent relationship between nursing mother and suckling infant. As a result, breastfeeding was dictated by the number of minutes infants suckled at their mother's breast as opposed to infant-led feeding. This rule-driven nature of breastfeeding has not led to positive outcomes for mothers or their infants. According to Penny Van Esterik, this biomedical influence negatively shapes breastfeeding, as it supports a commoditization of breastfeeding, which seeks to disembody the breast from mothers and present scientific evidence as solely objective (xv-xvi). Charlotte Faircloth also criticizes how this technocratic model of medicine attempts to gain a stronghold over women's bodies by continually discounting the role of maternal instincts (169).

Since 98.5 percent of women give birth in U.S. hospitals, the biomedical model plays a crucial role in how women are taught about breastfeeding with health campaigns that seek to educate women using the mantra "breast is best" (Hamilton 7). The current trend is to create an "objective truth" regarding the benefits of breastfeeding coupled with the belief that women need to be convinced to breastfeed, even though previous studies have found women to be well aware of these health benefits (Kukla 161). My research with first-time mothers supports these findings where 95 percent of the women in this study were familiar with the "breast is best" campaign and knowledgeable about the benefits of breastfeeding. Hanson argues that although medical science aspires to be neutral and objective, it cannot for the language we use at this moment is not value-free (13). Van Esterik believes that emphasis on the nutritional aspects of breastfeeding deviates from the broader picture of breastfeeding as a process heavily embedded in cultural, societal, and economic values (14; Scavenius et al. 678-79). In other words, breastfeeding consists of a complex interdependence between mother and child, which cannot be sectioned into a measurable and objective act. By examining breastfeeding as a process, researchers and mothers are better equipped to capture the transformative part of breastfeeding, encouraging a more equitable dialogue between mothers and healthcare professionals. Currently, medical professionals are the dominant voices in breastfeeding rhetoric, and this may play a role in the difficulties many women face trying to reach long-term breastfeeding goals that reflect these dominant voices as opposed to maternal ones. Due to this biomedical influence, healthcare initiatives focus on educating mothers to make the "right" choice—one narrowly defined by policymakers to encourage the breast-formula dichotomy with the resultant effect of mothers who feel pressure to nurse their infants according to arbitrary rules that disregard their own needs (Ma, "Critical Examination" 3). This chapter seeks to challenge the picture of breastfeeding shaped by healthcare initiatives by giving a voice to the nursing women because their narratives offer a broader understanding of breastfeeding that moves beyond infant feeding.

Methodology

One hundred and twenty first-time mothers were recruited from popular pregnancy websites, which hosted birth clubs or online support groups for women due the same month. Criteria for participation included being a first-time mother carrying a single child with no major complications, being eighteen years or older, and expressing a desire to breastfeed. These women were followed for three data waves consisting of the prenatal (twenty-eight to forty-two weeks of pregnancy), early postpartum (birth to three weeks) and late postpartum (four to twelve weeks) periods. They were asked to complete a series of quantitative measures and open-ended questions for a larger project examining breastfeeding beliefs. Although all race/ethnicities were represented, the women were primarily Caucasian with a mean age of twenty-eight with ages ranging between twenty-two and thirty-four. These women were primarily college educated with a median income of over $100,000.00, and the majority of them worked outside of the home. There was 8 percent attrition during the early postpartum (n = 110) and 35 percent for the late postpartum periods (n = 78). This research was approved by The Graduate Center of the City University of New York's Institutional Review Board, and participants' names were changed to a pseudonym in the final reporting.

Content analysis was used to examine open-ended responses to questions focusing on what mothers had learned from their journey into breastfeeding. This form of analysis is commonly used among researchers working with qualitative data and aims to classify written text into categories sharing the same meaning or themes (Cavanagh 5; Elo and Kyngas 108). The use of content analysis was a good fit with this study's aims, as it allowed the researchers to identify patterns among the participants' words that described the complex process of learning how to nurse their infants. Responses were read separately by two researchers, and recurrent themes were identified and tallied. Two overarching themes of confidence and resistance were revealed through the data. All data was collected using SurveyMonkey and encrypted using Secure Sockets Layer encryption technology, which is a cryptographic system securing the transmittance of private documents or information via the Internet.

Maternal Transformations in Confidence

Some of the biggest challenges facing women in breastfeeding consist of inconsistent or confusing information during the prenatal and postnatal periods, which pressure mothers to breastfeed without offering adequate support measures for personal breastfeeding goals that undermine maternal confidence (Cross-Barnet 1926; Nelson e17).

Our findings indicated that the mothers in this study overcame many of these challenges by relying on their infant's cues. Rather than embracing scientific mothering, these women realized their infants played an active role in breastfeeding. The move from breastfeeding as a scientific-based activity to one prioritizing informal cues from infants has the potential to buffer the current risk-reduction ideology that has developed in line with intensive-mothering strategies (Kukla 177; Wolf

600). Mothers who learn how to read infant feeding cues can change their experience of breastfeeding to be less fear or anxiety driven (e.g., breastfeeding to prevent disease, increase IQ, etc.) and more infant centred (Tedder 244-45). In this sense, breastfeeding facilitates an important maternal transformation that can increase a mother's confidence as she learns to read her infant's cues and is positively reinforced by her infant's response. In addition, infants benefit by having a mother who is sensitive to their nonverbal cues, which is their first form of communication. This may seem insignificant to the naïve or scientific eye, but it is the first step toward restructuring breastfeeding to centre the mother-infant dyad. Mothers who focused more on listening to their infants no longer viewed policymakers or medical professionals as the only authorities on breastfeeding. Maternal transformations in confidence became evident as these women acknowledged their own expertise in breastfeeding their infant, questioned outside experts, valued experiential learning, and realized the impact of their infant's responses to their care.

Trinity, mother to Cameron, stated how "moms know best" which acknowledges how maternal instincts and the amount of time mothers spend with their infants can make them an expert on their own child. Infant care during those first few weeks postpartum may seem tedious and never ending, but it provides the opportunity for a deeper connection with their infants, as compared to paediatricians who have far less contact. Addison, mother to Chloe, shared a similar sentiment: "Please don't preach about breastfeeding if you have never done it." She offers a critical view of breastfeeding, in which she recognizes the possibility that some experts may not have any practical experience. Stephanie, mother to Elijah said the following: "That they aren't experts unless they themselves have actually breast fed." Her sentiment echoes the same reaction as Addison where experiential breastfeeding holds a higher value than merely reading about the technical aspects. Many women first learn about breastfeeding using a generalized model that is believed to be true for all women, and when breastfeeding does not follow this model, they tend to doubt their ability to breastfeed. Evelyn, mother to Allison, realized that breastfeeding is a distinctive process encompassing individual differences, but it is often taught using a standardized, rule-driven model: "I've learned that it's different for everybody. I listened to lots of advice that does not apply to me and my baby." Learning in this top-down fashion also encourages women to rely on outside authorities—such as physicians, lactation consultants, and other experts—for the rules on how to successfully breastfeed. In reality, the reliance on teaching and surveillance from medical professionals has led to poor breastfeeding outcomes; the anxiety and stress from trying to abide by the rules have resulted in some women weaning their newborns sooner than they had hoped. Casting a critical eye toward breastfeeding experts led to more mothers listening and relying on their maternal instincts. These mothers began to view their own experiences as valid. Each of their responses show a greater appreciation of their lived experiences, and question whether authority figures are the only experts on breastfeeding. These discoveries led women to be more critical of the information they received from external sources and encouraged mothers to believe that the truth can come from within.

Kennedy, mother to Jenna, understood the value of relying on her instincts in finding solutions to her problems: "I learned to trust my instincts, or at least use sound logic and rational thinking instead of strictly adhering to the latest 'best advice.'" This pattern of behaviour was a common response during the late postpartum period. Although 89 percent of the sample did not consider themselves to be a breastfeeding expert, they made it clear that they were an expert on their own child. As Kennedy said, "I'm MY breastfeeding expert, I know what works for me. I can feel comfortable giving advice about what works for me to other moms. I guarantee I've done more research on normal, healthy breastfeeding and remedies to common breastfeeding issues in the past four months than my paediatrician has done in her life." Her response differentiates herself from the medical professionals whom she feels are less capable of helping breastfeeding women: "Doctors should stick to disorders and diseases and leave things alone that aren't broken." Her move away from medical professionals highlights her acceptance of the validity of her own experiences and listening to her inner voice. She was clear in how her decisions were idiosyncratic to her situation and may not work for other mothers. Surprisingly, her narrative was the first to view breastfeeding as a normative process between mother and child that does not require a physician's care. The biomedical model tends to define breastfeeding experts as limited to medical professionals, but Kennedy's narrative challenges this assumption and attempts to justify that the mother-infant dyad should be the primary expert. Multiple mothers shared similar responses, in which abiding by expert advice often left them more stressed about breastfeeding. In determining which knowledge is considered more valid, Faircloth found that a reliance on expert advice can encourage a risk-reduction mentality, which often increases parental paranoia and anxiety (23).

Molly, mother to Faith, was exhausted during the early postpartum period as her daughter nursed constantly, but she realized that her continuous nursing was the best way to get her milk to come in, which prompted her to see the use of schedules as arbitrary: "That there is no such thing as a schedule. In the beginning I was trying to follow "rules" it works better when you just relax." Her narrative hints at the stress of following rules that may not apply to the situation at hand, but can negatively affect a mother's milk supply. Her confidence was strong as a new mother and she attributed that to the reactions of her daughter: "I am a confident mother. I know what is best for my baby and I am assured by her responding to my care." Her last response reinforces the role of infant agency, as it provides support for the interdependence of maternal caregiving and infant response. This response also sheds light on the timing of breastfeeding classes, which are offered before an infant is born. Reading about breastfeeding or practising on a doll cannot capture the nuances of nursing an infant, as women viewed their infants as active participants in breastfeeding, which is often neglected in breastfeeding education. Breastfeeding classes may be more effective during the early postpartum period when mothers practise techniques on their own infants.

When Jennifer's daughter, Grace, was born, she experienced sore nipples but understood the importance of following her infant's schedule and trusting her instincts: "I've learned my baby's preferences, when she likes to eat, how and how much, when she's full, etc. I've also learned that there is a lot more to breastfeeding than I first thought! It can be a lot more difficult and painful than anyone tells you and at times frustrating." Women who learn to read their infant's cues often became more adept at mothering, which nurtures their maternal confidence (DiCarlo; Onwujuba and Baumgartner 205; Ma, *Eat at Mom's* 94; Ma, "Booby Traps" 14). Jennifer's narrative also exemplifies how maternal interpretation is critical to breastfeeding success, and highlights some of the unspoken truths regarding nipple pain. If she had relied only on the advice of medical professionals, she might have fallen for misleading information where experts often blame new mothers for not getting their infant to latch properly, resulting in sore nipples. Little is often said regarding how lip and/or tongue ties, small mouths, thrush, and pain medications given to mothers during labour can all affect infant latching and breastfeeding outcome. It is also common to advise mothers to nurse for twenty minutes on each breast to prevent sore nipples as opposed to employing effective strategies—such as applying pain-relieving sprays safe for nursing or using hydrogel dressings or glycerin gel therapy, which can alleviate the most common reason nursing women wean (Joanna Briggs Institute 2-3; Kent et al. 12256). In reality, newborns' mouths are small, and both parties are learning how to nurse. Soreness may continue for the first few weeks of nursing for some women; rather than acknowledge that reality to new mothers, medical experts often dismiss their pain. Although many women endured pain during their initial nursing experiences, they channelled this pain to transform how they viewed breastfeeding, particularly the mantra "breast is best."

Resisting Breast Is Best

There are two principles of the breast is best ideology that can unknowingly create obstacles for nursing mothers. The first problem is the assumption that educating women about the biomedical model of breastfeeding is sufficient for women to successfully breastfeed their infants. Rebecca Kukla points out that breastfeeding campaigns often fail to address the gap between knowing that the breast is best and actual breastfeeding behaviours (162). As mentioned earlier, 95 percent of the women in this study were familiar with the breast is best mantra, and even the mothers who weaned their infants still believed that breastfeeding was the optimal source of nutrition for their infants suggesting that they are educated about the benefits of breastfeeding. The second problem lies in how this ideology reinforces a narrow understanding of breastfeeding that encourages a dichotomous view where good mothers breastfeed and bad mothers do not. It is this mentality that incites conflict between militant nursing mothers and those who use formula (Faircloth 221). Most of the mothers in our study experienced difficulties during the early postpartum period, but those who strongly adhered to breast is best ideology were less resilient in adapting breastfeeding to suit their needs because they were more apt to force their experiences to match what they had originally learned during the prenatal period. Therefore, identifying ways women resisted the breast is best ideology may help new nursing mothers adopt a more flexible approach toward breastfeeding.

Angela, mother to Lucas, offered an example of resistance: "I still have questions and am learning new things all the time." Her narrative reveals an openness and acceptance toward not knowing everything about breastfeeding. Few individuals acknowledge how breastfeeding relies on a leap of faith because it is difficult to measure the amount of breastmilk an infant consumes through nursing. This ability to tolerate uncertainty is a critical aspect of resisting the biomedical model because it goes against the cookie-cutter model of breastfeeding education that stresses a single and proper way to breastfeed. Little is said about how infants learn to nurse in their own way, or how certain physical conditions (e.g., tongue-ties, lip ties, large breasts, suctioning at birth, etc.) can affect breastfeeding outcome. Mothers who experienced breastfeeding differently than how they had been taught felt that they were doing it wrong. These feelings reinforce the belief that there are correct and incorrect ways to nurse infants. Yet when nursing difficulties did ensue, mothers in the study exhibited resilience by creating their own model of breastfeeding that focused on their infant, similar to how previous mothers focused on infant cues. Miquelle, mother to Makayla, embraced a similar attitude: "There is a gradual process of balancing my body's production with my baby's needs and eating habits." Her words highlight how learning to breastfeed is a continual process that cannot be completed within a set period of time; it occurs gradually, which allows time for the body to attune to the infant's needs. In this sense, Miquelle understands how breastfeeding is a delicate balance between maternal and infant bodies. Her narrative further suggests that successful breastfeeding depends on fostering this interdependence while being open to different breastfeeding scenarios.

Reference to time in breastfeeding discourse is a common rhetoric where medical professionals often question when a mother's milk will come in, how long an infant should be nursed on each breast, what is considered an appropriate time to wean, why is a child cluster feeding, etc. All of these questions can undermine a mother's breastfeeding confidence (Tomori 39). Yet resistance shared by these two mothers also challenges the notion of time with regards to breastfeeding, which may buffer against maternal stress. Angela and Miquelle seemed more comfortable with the issue of time; they did not worry that there was a deadline for them to master breastfeeding. They both acknowledged the usefulness of experiential learning, as they simply nursed their infants and became sensitive to their reactions. In their narratives, they relied less on standardized information from published texts or experts, which can convey a linear progression with definitive rules—for example (e.g., to maintain your milk supply, you must feed the newborn every two hours for twenty minutes on each breast to prevent soreness). Instead, they used a more individualized outlook. These nursing women became more tolerant of the ambiguity that is characteristic of breastfeeding and receptive to the fact that breastfeeding can entail a continual state of learning with the confidence that as the needs of their bodies and infants change, so will their degree of knowledge to match those changes.

In our data, negotiating these grey areas became critical acts of resistance as mothers sought to breastfeed in ways that moved beyond black and white boundaries. Angela stated, "That breastfeeding is the best available method of feeding your child, but is not the only correct way." Her response breaks free from the breast is best ideology by acknowledging that flexibility in breastfeeding can result in a more positive and less anxiety-prone experience. Miquelle shared a similar view: "Breastfeeding, when possible, is the best choice for both mother and baby, offering health benefits to both and a bonding experience for mother and baby." Both women acknowledged the superiority of breastmilk over formula, but they exhibited flexibility in their decision-making strategies. Their wording implies that breastfeeding may not always be possible, yet their narratives do not vilify formula. Their words try to break free from the stress inherent in the dichotomous view between breastfeeding and the use of formula.

Natalie's and Christina's narratives also confirm the belief that breastfeeding should focus more on the individual mother and that the decision to nurse should be a personal one. Natalie, mother to Dawn, not only believed in the physical demands of breastfeeding but also discussed the psychological and emotional factors often neglected in breastfeeding literature: "It makes me think that people are promoting (pushing) breastfeeding on women who should be left to make their own very personal decisions." Her viewpoint suggests advocates pressure women to breastfeed under circumstances that may not be a good match to their own situations; she attempts to forefront the needs of the breastfeeding mother-infant dyad. Natalie also shared her expectations of breastfeeding: "I certainly hope that we get the hang of breastfeeding quickly and that neither of us finds it too taxing. I am trying to mentally prepare myself for a variety of outcomes so as to not be disappointed in expecting perfection." Her use of the word "perfection" is striking because it still reflects a right and wrong way to breastfeed. The strive toward perfection often leaves mothers little room to negotiate their mothering style and method of infant feeding, which often results in a deep sense of guilt and failure. Mothers in our sample experienced anxiety when breastfeeding did not match their prenatal expectations. Natalie's experience can teach women that breastfeeding can occur in a myriad of ways for both mother and infant and they have a hand in shaping their own breastfeeding realities to suit their individual needs. Subscribing to the breast is best ideology can negatively affect women's experiences of breastfeeding, but when mothers resisted this view, they learned how to think outside of the current boundaries of breastfeeding, which fostered flexibility in their thinking.

Christina, mother to Colin, shared a distinct outlook highlighting how normalization of breastfeeding can foster flexibility in thinking beyond the breast is best. She discussed how her decision to breastfeed was not based on researching its benefits, as compared to many of the mothers in this study. She continued to state how little she knew about breastfeeding; she had only read only one book, and could not ask her mother for advice for she had not been breastfed. Even though Christina had less formal preparation than the majority of the women in this study, she shared an important insight: "I live in Turkey, and they are very pro-breastfeeding here. My paediatrician and OB/GYN and the nurses at the hospital were very helpful. I have never seen a lactation consultant about breastfeeding." This cultural component may play a critical role in the normalization of and success in breastfeeding. Creating an accepting social atmosphere can be a crucial factor in breastfeeding success.

Nursing in public was a common concern for the mothers in our study, but if nursing is not readily accepted as a normative form of infant feeding, how can children and adults learn what is considered to be normative? Suzie Blake, an Australian artist and photographer, sought to challenge the current images of breastfeeding in the media (e.g., nursing supermodels or actresses) by creating a realistic photo series of nursing mothers called "What Does Breastfeeding Look Like?" (Willard). For new nursing mothers to be exposed to images of daily and realistic images of breastfeeding can be a powerful form of resistance for these women, as they challenge society's robust notions that breastfeeding should be hidden from the public eye. Living in a pro-breastfeeding culture may have influenced Christina's statement: "I believe that 'breast is best' depends on the person, what is right for some is not right for others." which suggests a subjective nature of how one defines what is "best." For some mothers, the breast is not always best, and breastfeeding should not be a measure of any mother's worth. Many first-time mothers fall into the trap of intensive mothering and aim to be the perfect mother under the false assumption that there is only one correct way to breastfeed. Faircloth finds that this aspect of intensive mothering—where breastfeeding is viewed as natural and all women share an innate capacity to enjoy breastfeeding—may contribute to feelings of failure when individualized breastfeeding experiences prove to be difficult and painful (168). The combination of intensive mothering and narrow views of breastfeeding as all-or-nothing fuels the dichotomy between breast and formula because if a mother cannot breastfeed, she believes that her only alternative is to wean and formula feed.

Shortly after giving birth, Christina admitted that she was having a difficult time; she worried about her milk supply and making sure her son had enough to eat. There were times when her son used her as a human pacifier and the only way to console him was to nurse him for hours on end: "I learned that babies are used to being fed constantly in the womb, and when they go through a growth spurt they can feed constantly. It just helps increase your supply." Her response normalizes cluster feedings and growth spurts, as she looks upon them in a positive manner, where continuous nursing would increase her supply. Rather than attribute the hours spent nursing to an insufficient milk supply, she interprets her son's actions in a normative fashion and focuses on how these long feedings may lead to a positive outcome. Living in a place where nursing is normalized may foster this flexibility in thinking, which can contribute to a more positive sense of corporeality as opposed to a faulty maternal body that produces insufficient milk. Many mothers viewed breast is best as a generalized rule that applied to all mothers and infants with little flexibility. Breastfeeding is more complicated than a dichotomous experience of pros and cons, as the nursing relationship between mother and child can go through a wide gamut of changes. When women's personal experiences differed from their formal education, the manner in which they were taught might have primed them to blame their own bodies as well as judge other mothers harshly as opposed to criticizing a faulty breastfeeding paradigm or seeking alternative approaches.

Conclusion

These narratives present an empowering and transformative view of breastfeeding. Cecília Tomori supports different methodological approaches in studying the embodied nature of breastfeeding as a way to examine the social implications of the nursing mother-infant dyad, which may encourage dialogue focusing on the specific needs of women (242). Breastfeeding in this manner can transform how women value their maternal instincts, embrace being an expert on their child, and gain confidence that their body will transcend any nursing challenge. The commonalities shared among this set of nursing mothers provide hope that breastfeeding can move beyond the narrow definitions espoused by medical professionals and experts so that women may break free from the surveillance of those in power and breastfeed according to their own needs and those of their infants. As women embrace the uniqueness of their breastfeeding experiences and the flexible nature of infant-feeding choices, this heightened sense of empowerment and confidence can help buffer the divide continuing to separate mothers. In highlighting the experiences of this sample of first-time mothers, we find breastfeeding to be on the cusp of becoming more than a mere method of infant feeding. By focusing on maternal transformations, we can create a new breastfeeding rhetoric that is not solely produced by the medical community but one that embodies the needs of nursing mothers. With advanced medical science and technology, it is easy to forget that breastfeeding begins and ends with a mother and her infant. Sometimes the advent of so-called experts results in self-doubt, which makes women question the embodied knowledge inherent in their bodies. Yet the most important people in breastfeeding are not policymakers, physicians, or lactation consultants but the mother-infant dyad. Focusing on maternal transformations through breastfeeding is an essential step toward this critical change because empowered mothers can change the world.

Works Cited

Blake, Suzie. What Does Breastfeeding Look Like? *Suzie Blake,* 2015, www.suzieblake.com/what-does-breastfeeding-look-like/. Accessed 23 July 2018.

"Breastfeeding Report Card, Progressing Toward National Breastfeeding Goals: United States, 2016." *Centers for Disease Control and Prevention,* 2016, www.cdc.gov/breastfeeding/pdf/2016breastfeedingreportcard.pdf. Accessed 23 July 2018.

Cavanagh, Stephen. "Content Analysis: Concepts, Methods and Applications." *Nurse Researcher,* vol. 4, no. 3, 1997, pp. 5-16.

Cross-Barnet, Caitlin, et al. "Long-Term Breastfeeding Support: Failing Mothers in Need." *Maternal and Child Health Journal,* vol. 16, no. 9, 2012, pp. 1926-32.

DiCarlo, Cynthia F, et al. "Infant Communicative Behaviors and Maternal Responsiveness." *Child and Youth Care Forum,* vol. 43, no. 2, 2013, pp. 195-209.

Eidelman, Arthur I., et al. "Breastfeeding and the Use of Human Milk." *Pediatrics,* vol. 129, no. 3, 2012, pp. e827-e841.

Elo, Satu, and Helvi Kyngas. "The Qualitative Content Analysis Process." *Journal of Advanced Nursing,* vol. 62, no. 1, 2008, pp. 107-115.

Faircloth, Charlotte. *Militant Lactivism?: Attachment Parenting and Intensive Motherhood in the UK and France.* Berghahn, 2013.

Hamilton, Brady, et al. "Births: Final Data for 2014." *National Vital Statistics Reports,* vol. 64, no. 12, 2015, pp. 1-64.

Hanson, Clare. *A Cultural History of Pregnancy. Pregnancy, Medicine and Culture, 1750-2000.* Palgrave, 2004.

"Healthy People 2020." *Office of Disease Prevention and Health Promotion,* Healthy People 2020. U.S. Department of Health and

Human Services, 2014, www.healthypeople.gov/. Accessed 23 July 2018.

Joanna Briggs Institute. "The Management of Nipple Pain and/or Trauma Associated with Breastfeeding." *Australian Nursing Journal*, vol. 17, no. 2, 2009, pp. 32-35.

Kent, Jacqueline, et al. "Nipple Pain in Breastfeeding Mothers: Incidence, Causes and Treatments." *International Journal of Environmental Research and Public Health*, vol. 12, no. 10, 2015, pp. 12247-63.

Kukla, Rebecca. "Ethics and Ideology in Breastfeeding Advocacy Campaigns." *Hypatia*, vol. 21, no. 1, 2006, pp. 157-80.

Ma, Catherine. "A Critical Examination of Breastfeeding Education: A Qualitative Analysis of How First Time Mothers Learn About Breastfeeding." *The Journal of Mother Studies*, vol. 1, 2016, pp. 1-23.

Ma, Catherine. "Booby Traps: How Breastfeeding Promotional Campaigns Undermine Maternal Breastfeeding Efforts." *Society for Public Health Education's (SOPHE) 65th Annual Meeting, Discovery 2014: New Health Education Strategies, Connections and Ideas*, 21 March 2014, Hyatt Regency Baltimore Inner Harbor, Baltimore, MD. Conference Presentation.

Ma, Catherine. "*Eat at Mom's: Critiquing and Rebuilding the Breastfeeding Paradigm.*" Dissertation. The Graduate Center of the City University of New York, 2013.

Nelson, Antonia, M. "A Metasynthesis of Qualitative Breastfeeding Studies." *Journal of Midwifery and Women's Health*, vol. 51, no. 2, 2006, pp. e13-e20.

Palmer, Gabrielle. *The Politics of Breastfeeding. When Breasts Are Bad for Business*. Pinter and Martin, 2009.

Scavenius, Michael, et al. "In Practice, the Theory is Different: A Processual Analysis of Breastfeeding in Northeast Brazil." *Social Science and Medicine*, vol. 64, no. 3, 2007, pp. 676-88.

Tedder, Jan. "The Roadmap to Breastfeeding Success: Teaching Child Development to Extend Breastfeeding Duration." *The Journal of Perinatal Education*, vol. 24, no. 4, 2015, pp. 239-48.

Tomori, Cecília. *Nighttime Breastfeeding. An American Cultural Dilemma*. Berghahn, 2015.

Willard, Laura. "23 Breastfeeding Photos that Convey the Perfectly Imperfect Reality of Nursing." *Upworthy*, 2015, www.upworthy.com/23-breastfeeding-photos-that-convey-the-perfectly-imperfect-reality-of-nursing. Accessed 23 July 2018.

Wolf, Joan B. "Is Breast Really Best? Risk and Total Motherhood in the National Breastfeeding Awareness Campaign." *Journal of Health Politics, Policy and Law*, vol. 32, no. 4, 2007, pp. 595-636.

Van Esterik, Penny. "Foreword." *Ethnographies of Breastfeeding: Cultural Contexts and Confrontations*, edited by Tanya Cassidy and Abdullahi El Tom, Bloomsbury Academic, 2015, pp. xv-xxiii.

Chapter Twelve

Muriel Rukeyser: "In the Body's Ghetto"

Laura Major

"Experiences taken into the body, and poetry is what is produced. And life is what is produced."—Muriel Rukeyser, *The Life of Poetry*

Muriel Rukeyser (1913-1980) in the above epigraph links the production of poetry to the production of life, and both are connected to the body. In these brief words, Rukeyser recognizes the intricate and complicated relationship between experience, the body, the creation of poetry, and the creation of life. Rukeyser reimagines in diverse ways the transformative effect of pregnancy and childbirth on the embodied self, and also what it means to birth and write babies and poems. She does not paint a rosy picture of pregnancy and childbirth; rather, she tackles and attempts to resolve the issues at stake in such a reimagining—the childbirth metaphor, embodiment, pregnant subjectivity, and intersubjectivity—while she pays attention to language and form in her poetry. By childbirth metaphor, I mean the comparison of giving birth to creative output; by embodiment, I mean the influence of the body on the mind; by pregnant subjectivity, I mean the unique experience of the pregnant subject in which the boundaries between self and other break down; and by intersubjectivity, I mean the interrelations between self and other.

Muriel Rukeyser wrote during the period spanning the ascent of Modernism and its backlash. Her work predates then corresponds to the mis of the women's movement. Rukeyser certainly had no "women's tradition of poetry" from which to draw, nor was it acceptable then to discuss the body, maternity, and sexuality. She was a groundbreaker or, in the words of Adrienne Rich, a "beginner," who enabled later women poets to turn to their bodies in their poetry. She was a "beginner" in the same way as Whitman and Dickenson were beginners: "They are openers of new paths, those who take the first steps, who therefore can seem strange and "dreadful" to their place and time" (Rich 62). Indeed, Rukeyser was deeply influenced by Whitman in numerous ways; one of which was the connection between the body and poetry, with Whitman being seen as the self-proclaimed "poet of the body" ("Song of Myself"). For both Whitman and Rukeyser, "resistance to conservative thinking is an embrace of the body in its complexity" (Barnat 105).

Rich laments the fact that Rukeyser's achievement has not been truly appreciated, despite her truly groundbreaking work: "Most of her work is out of print. Poets speak of her but she is otherwise barely known" (69).[1] Poet Anne Sexton similarly sums up Rukeyser's influence by calling her "mother of us all."[2] Sharon Olds, another poet of the body, reports she learned three things from Muriel Rukeyser: "Write about what they tell you to forget, write about what they tell you to forget, write about what they tell you to forget" (Garner). Rukeyser explicitly refers to the bodily experience of pregnancy and childbirth as falling into this category. Although her personal poems dealing with these experiences are my primary focus, it is important to note that Rukeyser, as a political and social activist (who was on file with the FBI), saw poetry also as functioning as a mode of social and political protest.

Rukeyser was a poet of the self who recognized connections to others comprise that self. Rukeyser was engrossed with these conn-ections and made her poems "for others unseen and unborn" in order to "reconcile ... ourselves with each other/ourselves with ourselves" ("Poem"). Rukeyser also collapses the procreation-creation binary in ways allowing for the emergence and coexistence of poetic and maternal subjectivity. She demonstrates that only by claiming the "birthwrite," the ability and right to both write and birth, can pregnant subjectivity successfully emerge.

Muriel Rukeyser understood the act of revision or reimagination as a poetic task: "People assume we have to have national and paternal civilizations, but that has to be re-imagined. The woman poet seems to me the sign of it" (qtd. in Speare 2162). More significantly, she undertook this task in her poetry by critically reimagining some of the dominant myths and tales of Western civilization. In "Miriam: The Red Sea," for example, she rewrites the splitting of the red sea from Miriam's perspective, whereas the poem "Ms. Lot" tells the story of Lot's daughters in their voices. Rukeyser also rewrote many Greek myths in women's voices, challenging the authority of these tales in "Waiting for Icarus," "Myth," and "In Hades-Orpheus."

Perhaps the most powerful example of Rukeyser's poetical reimagination of myth is "The Poem as Mask," which not coincidentally deals with the poet's experience of childbirth. The memory of giving birth and the telling of this experience provoke a radical revision not only of myth but also of the poet's previous reading of myth and writing of poetry. This is a poem about giving birth, about constructing an unmasked self, and about writing poetry. Although it is the most powerful, "The Poem as Mask" is not the only poem that Rukeyser wrote about childbearing. In addition to "Nine Poems for an Unborn Child," she used birth imagery extensively in other poems to describe creativity.

Rukeyser challenged the tradition silencing the experiences of pregnancy and childbirth. In a review of Charlotte Marletto's book *Jewel of our Longing*, Rukeyser described the literary situation until 1949 regarding childbirth poetry as follows: " There is no poetry of birth in the literature that reaches us. In our own time we can count the poems on our fingers; there is a great blank behind us, in our classic and religious literature. There we might expect to find the clues to human process and common experience" (qtd. in Eisenberg 185)." In this same piece, Rukeyser goes on to state that "In the books about the artist ... there is absolutely no allowance made for the possibility of the woman artist" (qtd. in Goldensohn 128). Rukeyser, thus, implicitly links the poetic silence regarding childbirth to the exclusion of the woman artist or poet. She sets out to challenge the cultural discourse separating procreation from creation both because it views pregnancy and childbirth as inappropriate subject matter for poetry and because it sees childbearing and rearing, and not writing, as the tasks of women. This challenge demands a double deconstruction: the writing of childbirth poetry as a refutation of the claim that "childbirth" and "poetry" cannot co-exist, and the metapoetical collapse of the dichotomy between the experience of pregnancy and childbirth and the metaphor of pregnancy and childbirth.

Nine Poems for the Unborn Child

Rukeyser's "nine poems for the unborn child," which is a sequence that gradually works out the mother's relationship to her fetus, precedes the more symbolic exploration of pregnancy in "The Poem as Mask." The "nine poems" sequence, written during Rukeyser's pregnancy in 1947, betrays a certain distance from the body; we detect the very masks that she later tries to throw off in "The Poem as Mask." Yet in 1947, before any political feminist movement existed, writing poetry about pregnancy, birth, and breastfeeding especially as a single mother—or as she called herself in "The Speed of Darkness," a "bastard mother"—was truly pioneering. It was perhaps this groundbreaking nature of her poetry that inspired the titles of two important early anthologies of women's poetry; Louise Bernikow's *The World Split Open* and Florence Howe's *No More Masks* both take their titles from Rukeyser poems.

Each section in "nine poems" represents a month of the gestation period, and the poet's relationship to her fetus changes and evolves with her growing body. In the first poem about the "childless years alone without a home," words describing insufficiency abound: "alone," "little to give, and always less to take," "loss," "hardly-moving." The sense that she is incomplete without a child sets the stage for the second poem in which: "They came to me and said, 'There is a child.'" The lines following this announcement link her knowledge of being with child to her image-making facilities: "Fountains of images broke through my land. / My swords, my fountains spouted past my eyes / And in my flesh at last I saw." Not only does her awareness of her pregnancy unleash "fountains of images," but "at last" these images come from her "flesh," her bodily experience. No longer do her eyes exclusively render images: her flesh, her body, has become the site of sight. That Rukeyser takes the line "and in my flesh at last I saw" from the *Book of Job*—"in my flesh shall I see God" (Job 19:26)—may impart religious significance to her pregnancy while recognizing the potential for suffering, the theme of Job, in maternity.

Poem III contains a remarkable description of what is going on inside her womb, for it corresponds to the ultrasound images to which we today have access, but certainly not in 1947:

> The wave of smooth water approaches on the sea-
> Surface, a live wave individual
>
> Linking, massing its color. Moving, is struck by wind
> Ribbed, steepened, until the slope and ridge begin;
> Comes nearer, brightens. Now curls, its vanishing
> Hollows darken and disappear; now high above
> Me, the scroll, froth, foam of the overfall.

The wave that she describes above becomes the fetal movement or quickening described in poem IV: "The waves are changing, they tremble from waves of waters / To other essentials." The poet is still focused on her own reactions to her pregnancy rather than on the fetus, which she describes through repeated use of the words "my" and "me"—the effect of this quickening on her. It is as if the movements within her have an effect on her sense of self, as if the quickening makes her aware of her own bodily existence. This brings to mind Sara Ruddick's discussion of the activity of waiting, which engages the pregnant woman's moral, intellectual, and relational capacities (42). The waves become "waves of light / And wander through *my* sleep and through *my* waking, / And through *my* hands and over *my* lips and over *Me*" (my emphasis).

Already in poem V, she moves from a focus on self to an exploration of the other—the fetus inside her. She is, however, unsure of the nature of this other and asks: "Who is in the dim room? Who is there?" In poem VI, although her question remains unanswered, she is thrown into an awareness of the separate existence of her and her child. In the first moment she understands that this baby, while also a part of her, is truly other or separate from herself, Rukeyser describes how they (supposedly the doctors) "came to me and said, 'If you must choose / Is it yourself or the child?'" Her response to this existential question portrays the shock of her realization that the radical separation of the other from the self in birth brings one to a heightened state of being, with the possibilities of death and life intricately bound: "Laughter I learned / In that moment, laughter and choice of life." This laughter betrays not only shock but also a paralysis: How does one choose between one's own life and the life of another who is not quite yet a person?

The end of poem VI points us to her choice: "I saw a child. I saw / A red room, the eyes, the hands, the hands and eyes." The thought of choosing makes her aware for the first time of the materiality of her baby. No longer does she describe the waves, winds, and waters of the previous poems, but the physical matter of "the eyes, the hands, the hands and eyes." She has to repeat these words in order to internalize their meaning. Rukeyser frames the words "I saw a child" with spaces on either side to highlight the significance of this awareness; "seeing" or imagining her child as child for the first time is a momentous realization.

Having experienced this realization, Rukeyser in poem VII focuses solely on this child addressing him for the first time; this poem contains no trace of Rukeyser's lyric "I." She structures the poem by repeating four times the words "You will enter the world" at the beginning of every second line of the first eight lines. This repetition seems to function to convince the poet that this child will indeed leave her body and enter the world. The last words of poem VII—"you will enter the world"—cement her realization. She needs this cement, as the world that she describes is a fearsome place "where death by fear and explosion/ Is waited" and "where various poverty / Makes thin the imagination and the bone." It is a world of language where language has destructive potential: "You will enter the world which eats itself / Naming faith, reason, naming love, truth, fact." To come into the world of language is to come into a world where nothing is experienced purely as in the womb, but where language, definition, and culture mediate our every emotion and experience. The poet intimates that it may be preferable that "you in your dark lake" remain sheltered inside, but she accepts the inevitability of birth and its implications for the child in the spondaic heavy closing statement: "you will enter the world."

Now that the poet has recognized the other as other, she returns in poem VIII to her self, or, more accurately, to the self-other pregnant unit. Indeed the mother and child are completely implicated in each other:

> Child who within me gives me dreams and sleep,
> Your sleep, your dreams; you hold me in your flesh
> Including me where nothing has included
> Until I said: I will include, will wish
> And in my belly be a birth....

Dreams of an unborn child move through my dreams.

The child's dreams move through hers; she holds him in her flesh, and he holds her in his. Mother and child, separate but connected, exist in this poem in a not quite real world, where sunlight (versions of the word "sun" are repeated four times in this section), dreams (appearing five times) and waves (three times) abound. This idyllic symbiosis is a temporary utopian prelude to the birth, which will introduce the child into the unsympathetic, cold world Rukeyser describes in the previous stanza.

The ninth poem is the climax of the sequence in the same way that the ninth month is the climax of the pregnancy and her symbolic understanding of it. This final poem returns to a focus on the mother, especially emphasizing her conception of her pregnant body. Being without child she had "known in [herself] hollow bodiless shade." Rukeyser connects the hollowness to being "lost and lost" and the pregnancy to "at last" being found. The following run-on line with its curious syntax implies that the pregnant body is a home not only for the growing fetus but also for the mother: "Praise that the homeless may in their bodies be / A house that time makes, where the future moves / In his dark lake." Homeless describes the prepregnant state, recalling the very first line of the first poem: "The childless years alone without a home." Rukeyser offers praise that pregnancy makes herself and, as the plural indicates, other women "in their bodies be," or experience their bodies as home. This is, of course, pregnancy felt in and through the body. Of course, as the run-on line indicates, the praise is also directed to their bodies' housing of the fetus or the future: "in their bodies be a house." Rukeyser closes the poem with the poignant hope: "To live, to write, to see my human child." The poignancy results from the underlying fear she may die during childbirth. Even when confronting this fear of the bodily consequences of giving birth, her hope she will continue writing precedes even her hope to see her human child. Here, she announces her identity as poet will not be compromised by her motherhood.

I would have liked to conclude this short analysis by saying Rukeyser's hope, as expressed in "nine poems for an unborn child," that her creative and procreative functions could co-exist in harmony was fulfilled. But Rukeyser referred to the first ten years after giving birth as "the intercepted years," and as Kate Daniels tells us, "the dramatic and immediate decrease in her literary production testifies to the labour-, time-, and energy-intensive project of childrearing" (xiii). The tension between being a mother (especially a single mother like Rukeyser) and being a poet exists; no amount of theoretical deconstructing of the divisions between these realms can erase this tension. It is, however, a productive tension that can produce and enhance poetry.[3] To reimagine the pregnant and birthing self does not demand a positive representation. The recognition of the pain and difficulties involved is central for a real and an unsentimental confrontation with these states of being. Emmanuel Levinas presented pregnancy as the ultimate suffering for the other and, therefore, the very basis of ethical relations (75). In "The Poem as Mask," Rukeyser goes even further in reimagining a pregnant and birthing self, whose torn, split-open nature enhances rather than detracts from the reimagination.

The Poem as Mask

The subtitle of "The Poem as Mask"—"Orpheus"—refers not only to the myth of Orpheus but also to Rukeyser's poetic rendering of that myth. In her long 1949 poem "Orpheus," Rukeyser internalizes the intention of the original myth and celebrates it; she describes how Orpheus, the greatest musician alive, was torn to pieces by the Bacchantes and then miraculously made whole. His body parts are reunited so that he can sing eternally. Rukeyser thought highly of this poem constructed as a court masque; it is one of the only poems on which she expounds in her prose meditation *The Life of Poetry* (1949). Rachel DuPlessis explains that "the singer as sacred, the fragments of the human reunited as the divine, the transcendent experience of healing and power combined in the figure of Orpheus are motifs with great resonance for Rukeyser" (293). Yet twenty years later, she would rewrite her own rewriting of the Orpheus myth in "The Poem as Mask, Orpheus."

"The Poem as Mask" is then a double reimagining: a rewriting of the myth but, more significantly, a rewriting of her own conception of this myth and of myth in general. But it is also explicitly a reimagining of her self. The event of childbirth, or more accurately the memory of that event, changes her as reader of myth and of her self, enabling a radically transformed reading and writing experience. The revision of myth is a complex process: myth is not a mere story, but one that is retold until it comes to be accepted as truth. Moreover, it becomes a part of our language system (Lauter 2). Once a myth is in place, Estella Lauter explains, "it is nearly impossible to dislodge it by exclusively rational means. It must be replaced by another equally persuasive story or symbol" (1). To revise a myth then is to revise deep levels of individual and cultural consciousness. That Rukeyser displaces the Orpheus myth with her personal experience of childbirth underscores the potency and symbolic meaning of that experience.

Rukeyser opens the poem by criticizing her former celebration of the Orpheus myth; she acknowledges the masque was actually a mask:

> When I wrote of the women in their dances and wildness, it
> was a mask,
> on their mountain, gold-hunting, singing in orgy
> it was a mask; when I wrote of the god,
> fragmented, exiled from himself, his life, the love gone down
> with song,
> it was myself, split open, unable to speak, in exile from myself.

Rukeyser recognizes the image of Orpheus torn apart was merely a vehicle for her own feelings, but instead of bringing her closer to her authentic experience of pain, the metaphor only removed her from what she wanted to express. The self that appears in the last line of this stanza is an alienated, a conflicted, and a silenced self: "it was myself, split open, unable to speak, in exile from myself." The structure of these lines links this self to the mask. By repeating the syntax of the first lines—"when I wrote of ... it was a mask"—and substituting "mask" with "myself"—"when I wrote of ... it was myself"—Rukeyser establishes a masked self. The speaker recognizes the mask and her thorough identification with Orpheus perpetuate the exile and inhibition of her voice. Rukeyser may also be making a statement against the principles of High Modernism that exalted the use of the mask and decried the personal. Modernist poetry, she seems to state, alienates the poet from herself.

The poet realizes she has mistakenly, and too wholly, identified with a mythical figure who cannot possibly represent her experience; her identification with Orpheus in the poem "Orpheus" is not sufficiently grounded in a strong conception of self so as to enable recognition of a separate female embodied self. This knowledge and the need to completely differentiate her experience from his bring her to a momentary obliteration of any identification with the god.

To terminate the alienation from herself an to get closer to her self, she strips away the masking images and the object of her paralyzing identification: "There is no mountain, there is no god." She reveals in their stead her own experience: ... there is memory / of my torn life, myself split open in sleep, the rescued child beside me among the doctors, and a word of rescue from the great eyes." The rebirth of the god in "Orpheus" cannot convey the experience of the real birth of her own child. Orpheus's fragmentation cannot describe her experience of being torn and being cut open in surgery. The healing of Orpheus is nothing in comparison to the rescue of the infant from her womb. Moreover, the experience of becoming a mother serves to metaphorically describe her life far more authentically than myth. Hers is a separate miracle, so vivid and unique in her mind that it cannot be sharpened by the use of myth but only blunted through a mask.

Rukeyser also understands that concealing under the symbols of myth the unpoetic, unaesthetic aspects of womanhood such as giving birth, or being "split open," only perpetuates their taboo nature. Rukeyser insists on writing all aspects of experience and especially the experience of maternity. Indeed, she addresses the dearth of poetic representation of these experiences: "Few of the women writing poetry have made more than a beginning in writing about birth.... And the young men in poetry seem, for the great part, to suffer so form the fear of birth that we have a tabu [*sic*] deep enough in our culture to keep us ever from speaking of it as a tabu" (qtd. in Daniels, xvi). In reaction against this taboo, Rukeyser pledges in her iconoclastic line following the brief description of her surgery: "No more masks! No more mythologies!"

The description of her actual experience of giving birth is sparse, perhaps because the speaker's account of being "split open in sleep" is a description of a Caesarean section performed under anesthesia. Rukeyser gave birth by Caesarean section, only to wake up and discover that an unauthorized hysterectomy had also been performed. In any event, in this poem the actual occasion of giving birth is secondary to its symbolic meaning. "Memory," as invoked by Rukeyser, involves a reinterpretation of the past in the present. Memory can never produce a replica of the actual event especially when the event in question is an operation under anesthesia. Thus, the importance lies in how memory records the interpretation of this experience and invests this interpretation with symbolic meaning (Smith and Watson 16). Her personal memory of the moment that she became a mother catalyzes the radical change in her conception of self, of myth, and of poetry. Her awesome feeling of rescue—the word is mentioned twice in this stanza—combined with the proximity of death and life, fertility and sterility, wounding and healing, brings her to a transformational experience of her body, an experience of the most existential states of being.

The image of being "split open" surfaces twice in this poem, each time with a different meaning. When Rukeyser first describes the feeling of being "split open," she is describing a feeling of alienation, of being "unable to speak, in exile from myself;" the second use of "split open" renders the very physical experience of Caesarean section. Neither use has a positive connotation. "Splitting open," however, is an image of great resonance for Rukeyser. Her numerous uses of this image, which significantly often appear together with birth imagery, offer other perspectives on what it means to be split open. Although Ruth Porrit is correct in noting that Rukeyser is not completely consistent in her use of this image (180), perhaps this inconsistency is inherent in the image: "splitting open" after all defies unity, wholeness, and consistency while invoking fragmentation and multiplicity.

"Splitting open" appears in one of Rukeyser's most famous lines in her poem "Kathe Kollwitz." There she asks: "What would happen if one woman told the truth about her life? / The world would split open." This poem is important not only because of its expression of Rukeyser's "splitting open" vision, but also because of Rukeyser's identification with Kollwitz, a German artist and activist who rebelled against myths of aggression and instead created mythical mother figures (Lauter 14-15). Kollwitz's reimagination of myth exemplifies for Rukeyser the heroic act of attempting to change the world through art. That Kollwitz replaced patriarchal myths with matriarchal ones further strengthens Rukeyser's argument that truth telling comes from the experience of the maternal body.

In this light, Rukeyser's body, "split open" for the delivery of her child, comes to signify the connection between the individual telling the truth about life, and changing the world. A woman telling the truth about her experience in highly personal moments, such as childbirth, breaks up the unity and harmony of cultural myths. The act of splitting open or deconstructing myths shows them to be not eternal, untouchable truths, but simply texts without a highly privileged status. Moreover, once the myth has been split open, once a taboo has been broken, and once the deconstruction process has been set in motion, the possibilities for reimagining, reconstructing, and for retelling new versions and new truths—and for material change—are endless. For Rukeyser, the connection between the individual realm ("What would happen if one woman told the truth about her life?") and the social realm ("The world would split open") is essential. Rukeyser believed that to have an impact on history, one must first reach one's personal history ("there is memory / of my torn life"), since the "personal unconscious" is part of a "collective unconscious" (DuPlessis 289).

Rukeyser takes the "splitting open" image even further in "Recovering":

> Darkness arrives
> splitting the mind open
>
> Something again
>   is beginning to be born.

The poet describes the process of imagination in which the splitting open of the mind precedes the birth of "something," of a poem. This "something" is progeny of the mind and recalls the typical male use of the childbirth metaphor, in which the poet gives birth to poems from his mind. But the "splitting open" image throughout Rukeyser's poetry, as opposed to in an isolated poem, ruptures the mind-body dichotomy. The process of birthing described above is analogous to the way in which her body in "The Poem as Mask" had to be split open before her child could be born. These lines deepen our understanding of the moment of being split open as a moment of crisis, as darkness arriving, or as an invasive surgical intervention. In the end, the splitting open will yield the birth of child or of poem, "something" new, "something" with regenerative potential.

The vision of the interrelationship between splitting open, birth, poetry, and truth-telling climaxes in "The Speed of Darkness":

> I am he am I? Dreaming?
> I am the bird am I? I am the throat?
>
> A bird with a curved beak.
> It could slit anything, the throat-bird.
>
> Drawn up slowly. The curved blades, not large.
> Bird emerges wet being born.
> Begins to sing.

The speaker tentatively identifies herself, through questioning, as a newborn bird and as its throat—that is, as both the producer of the song, the means of singing, and the product of birth. In addition, as poet, she also gives birth to the bird/song by slitting herself open to emerge. This is a fusion of self/other, doing/done to, outside/inside images. Additionally, her poetic giving birth and being born are intricately linked to her actual childbearing experience; the "curved blades," as Jan Johnson Drantell argues, may refer to the surgical blade that performed her own Caesarean section (141). And this curved blade, which is also the curved beak of the bird, "could slit anything." Slitting appears here as a version of splitting open. In these short lines, Rukeyser fuses giving birth to child, to song, and to self so completely that the separations between these categories collapse.

Returning to "The Poem as Mask," we notice the last two lines of the poem revise her sweeping rejection: "No more masks! No more mythologies!" Indeed the final two lines return to myth and to the god, but it is a myth and god transformed. Paradoxically, by momentarily rejecting myth and its alienating truth status, the poet can grasp the poetic power of myth for the first time. The god now becomes a type of inspiring and enabling muselike figure: "Now for the first time, the god lifts his hand, / The fragments join in me with their own music." Her fragments are not unified as Orpheus was; rather, they remain fragments and form a new personal and cultural myth: "join in me with their own music." In "Orpheus" she claims, "All myths are within the body when it is most whole," whereas in "the Poem as Mask" the unwhole, split-open, and fragmented body is the site of authentic music. Each element of her "torn life" plays its own tune. The splitting open of the world by telling the truth creates poetry just as her physical experience of being split open yielded her child. Creation and procreation, however, are not only connected metaphorically but also in a concrete manner. In giving life by birthing (as opposed to Orpheus dying as a prelude to rebirth), her creative powers are unleashed to form "their own music" or poetry.

Endnotes

1 Although some symposia were held in 2013 to mark one hundred years since her birth, and some new articles have been published, this statement remains largely true today.

2 Sexton referred to Rukeyser in this way in a letter written to her on 1 November 1967.

3 Numerous examples attest to this fact; Sylvia Plath wrote her best poems while singlehandedly raising her small two children; Adrienne Rich wrote fine poetry in snatches between her three small boys'naps. Alicia Ostriker, Sharon Olds, Rita Dove, Toi Derricote, Lucille Clifton, Anne Sexton, and Audre Lorde are examples of other poets who experienced this tension, and used it to write poetry.

Works Cited

Barnet, Dara. "'Women and Poets see the Truth Arrive': Rukeyser and Whitman." *Studies in American Jewish Studies* 34.1 (2015): 96–116.

Daniels, Kate, editor. *Out of Silence: Selected Poems.* TriQuarterly Books, 1992.

Drantell Jan. "Or What's a Mother For?: Muriel Rukeyser as Mother/Poet." "*How Shall We Tell Each Other of the Poet?": The Life and Writing of Muriel Rukeyser,* edited by Anne F Herzog and Janet E Kaufman, St. Martin's, 1999, pp. 137-48.

DuPlessis, Rachel Blau. "The Critique of Consciousness and Myth in Levertov, Rich and Rukeyser." *Shakespeare's Sisters: Feminist Essays on Women Poets,* edited by Sandra Gilbert and Susan Gubar, Indiana University Press, 1979, pp. 281-300.

Eisenberg, Susan. "'Changing Waters Carry Voices': 'Nine Poems for the Unborn Child'." "*How Shall We Tell Each Other of the Poet?":The Life and Writing of Muriel* Rukeyser, edited by Anne F Herzog and Janet E Kaufman, St. Martin's, 1999, pp. 184-92.

Garner, Dwight. "Online Interviews with Sharon Olds." Modern American Poetry. www.english.illinois.edu/maps/poets/m_r/olds/onlineinterviews.htm. Accessed 8 Aug. 2018.

Goldensohn, Lorrie. "Our Mother Muriel." "*How Shall We Tell Each Other of the Poet?": The Life and Writing of Muriel Rukeyser*, edited by Anne F Herzog and Janet E Kaufman, St. Martin's, 1999, pp. 121-34.

Lauter, Estella. *Women as Mythmakers: Poetry and Visual Art by Twentieth-Century Women*. Indiana University Press, 1984.

Levinas, Emmanuel. *Otherwise Than Being or Beyond Essence*. Translated by, Alphonso Lingis, Duquesne University Press, 1998.

Olds, Sharon. "The Language of the Brag." *Satan Says*. Pittsburgh University Press, 1980.

Porrit, Ruth. "'Unforgetting Eyes': Rukeyser Portraying Kollwitz's Truth." "*How Shall We Tell Each Other of the Poet?": The Life and Writing of Muriel Rukeyser*, edited by Anne F Herzog and Janet E Kaufman, St. Martin's, 1999, pp. 163-83.

Rich, Adrienne. "Beginners." "*How Shall We Tell Each Other of the Poet?": The Life and Writing of Muriel Rukeyser*, edited by Anne F Herzog and Janet E Kaufman, St. Martin's, 1999, 62-69.

Rukeyser, Muriel. *The Collected Poems*. McGraw-Hill, 1978.

Rukeyser, Muriel. *Breaking Open*. Random House, 1973.

Speare, Cynthia Nanette. "Reimagined Myths of Muriel Rukeyser." MA Thesis. California State University, 1996.

Chapter Thirteen

Freedom to Labour–A Case Study on Childbirth Education and the Creation of Medical Choreographies

Katie Nicole Stahl-Kovell

In my research, I often hear participants lament about their inability to move their bodies off the hospital bed during their experiences of childbirth. In their own words: "I wasn't allowed to move" or "I was told I needed to be lying down in the bed" or "I wasn't told I had any other options." As a critical dance studies scholar and anthropologist, I ask how does a childbearing woman learn the technique of submission to medical authority prior to childbirth? In other words, how do pregnant women learn to have their childbearing bodies policed, ensuring conformity to the medical industrial complex? How do they then navigate these tight spaces of control—medical choreographies—to create their own choreographies of birth? Perhaps surprisingly to childbirth scholars and activists, I argue that childbirth education, especially hospital-sponsored, free-to-the-community classes, often run counter to a childbearing woman's bodily autonomy, whereas classes outside the hospital are designed to empower a woman's autonomy. These childbirth classes sponsored by hospitals frequently emphasize pain and teach mothers to expect their bodies to be dangerous to the baby and self. These classes can effectively prepare the pregnant body to relinquish control and be policed by medical authority. Yet although hospital-sponsored childbirth education classes can train the pregnant body to expect pain and to expect their body to be dangerous to the baby and self, during these classes women do find out what to expect of these medical choreographies. With that knowledge can become birth choreographers themselves, mobilizing movement as political action and finding fissures and cracks within seemingly ironclad medical choreographies.

Medical Choreographies of a Dangerous Kind—Theory and Methodology

Theory

This chapter addresses the impact childbirth education has on the childbearing body and evaluates how childbearing women respond to medical choreographies they learn in childbirth education. Medical choreographies are the speech acts and policies in action we can readily observe from any labour and delivery ward in a U.S. hospital. The intent of these choreographies is to de-mobilize a mother's and a baby's bodily autonomy. Expanding on Andre Lepecki's theory of choreopolicing from "Choreopolice and Choreopoitics: or, the task of the dancer," medical choreography, like police choreography, forces a standardization of mobility—in the case of the labour and delivery ward, standardization of care. Lepecki clarifies that police choreographies or choreopolicing imposes "a forced ontological fitting between pregiven movements, bodies in conformity, and pre-assigned places for circulation" (Lepecki 20). Conformity is key to a successful police and medical choreography. The entire purpose of both police and medical choreographies are to "de-mobilize political action by means of implementing a certain kind of movement that prevents any formation and expression of the political" (20). These movements implemented by doctors, nurses, and in this case study childbirth educators are created through the process of educating pregnant women what they are and are not allowed to do with their own bodies while delivering their baby in a hospital. In the case study that follows, we will encounter the educator weaving tight and, at times, suffocating medical choreographies that seemingly lead to dead ends, in which autonomy for mother and baby are nowhere to be seen except in the space in-between—the space where mother as dancer in this medical choreography learns to, echoing Lepecki's call, "claim kinetic knowledge on how to move towards freedom" and find a way amid these spaces of control to move both their and their baby's body politically (22).

It is difficult for women to move politically within the medical industrial complex in the United States because of the common construction of the female body as uncontrollable. In "Beyond Control: Body and Self in Women's Childbearing Narratives," Shannon Carter contends that popular media, social theory, and women themselves find their childbearing body to be "uncontrollable, uncontained, unbounded, unruly, leaky and wayward" (Carter 993). It is evident to see that medical choreography is put in place by medical professionals to treat the pregnant and childbearing body as a threatening and volatile being, especially during labour. Policing through the use of electronic fetal monitoring (EFM) despite its disproven efficacy, frequent cervical checks which risk the possibility of infection, and other technocratic means of control treat the childbearing body as something that needs to be controlled. My participants in this study searched for the fissures and cracks in this elaborate system of control throughout the childbirth education course as follows.

Medical choreographies are set in place to ensure a leaky, wayward childbearing body conforms to standardized care. These choreographies are dictated through hospital-sponsored childbirth education classes. Few scholars have evaluated childbirth education classes in the United States. Attendance for childbirth education classes is arguably on the decline, since pregnant people have access to massive amounts of free information through social media and online search engines. Childbirth education classes initially developed in the 1960s to combat maternal mortality and to assist with finding techniques for comfort during labour (Marin et al. 110). In more recent years, classes have come to assist in actual childbirth preparedness, informed decision making, and infant care (110-11). Most data on childbirth education classes comes from "Listening to Mothers"—three incredibly detailed national surveys on U.S. childbearing women's experiences. These surveys are devoted to improving healthcare from mothers and babies (9). The study found that every informant did not enrol in childbirth education classes due to cost and time. In their own words, "adding another source did not seem necessary" whey they "felt they were well-informed of the things that would and could happen during childbirth"

(109). Postpartum, their informants all expressed a lack of control over their birth experience and the authors argue that childbirth education classes could have enabled them to make informed decisions and bolster confidence in birth as a natural and normal process (111). Hospital-sponsored childbirth education, though, arguably teaches medical choreographies in order to control the volatile childbearing body under the guise of teaching pregnant folks about the birth process. Though the authors from "Listening to Mothers" argue that childbirth education does empower pregnant people to make informed decisions, learning medical choreographies is a much more complex act, teaching the pregnant person to expect to be policed, rather than simply empowering them to make their own autonomous decisions. Expanding on Jane Staton Savage's work on childbirth education, arguably "knowing does not diminish conflict surrounding the event and may even exacerbate it when not combined with learning skills to manage conflict" (Savage 10). The childbearing woman must learn at this juncture to not only understand and recognize medical choreographies, but to also negotiate for her and her baby's life through these uncomfortable and somewhat dangerous spaces of control. Childbirth education classes are sites where pregnant women can learn about medical choreographies and start to choreograph their own way through.

The choreopolitical task of the dancer and the childbearing woman is to always find a "way to move politically" amid spaces of control (Lepecki 20). But how do childbearing women find and activate the political in their movements in labour after taking childbirth education classes? They need to experiment with what fits best for their bodies and draw up a program, better known as a birth plan. In this particular childbirth education class that the case study explores below, the pregnant women were not encouraged whatsoever to write a birth plan. In other words, the educator wished them to submit to the preordained medical choreography. When a woman draws up a birth plan, she creates the political. In this world of control and as Lepecki explains regarding choreopolicing, the political moves "across agents, short-circuiting policed systems of obedience and command" through careful planning (22). This is where we see and bear witness to women in labour becoming birth choreographers. Pregnant women are not just participating as dancers within an elaborate medical choreography; rather, they are agents, figuring out how to subvert the conformity the medical industrial complex deems necessary. Dance studies scholar Anthea Kraut best explains that naming someone a choreographer assigns agency and premeditated calculation. Naming a childbearing woman a birth choreographer pushes back against the pervasive, masculinist, and misogynistic rhetoric driving U.S. maternal healthcare, which paints the birthing woman as a writing, animalistic creature who—without necessary medicalized interventions—is inconsolable and out of control.

Methodology

For this case study, I attended a childbirth education course with a pregnant participant, interviewed a doula who also attended the same course, interviewed a childbirth educator who previously taught the same course at the same location in the past, conducted one prenatal interview with the pregnant participant, and followed up with one postpartum interview with the participant within six weeks of her experience of labour. The participant signed her approval to participate in this study under the University of Riverside's Human Research Review Board and remains anonymous to protect her identity.

As a participant-observer in the childbirth education course, I told the educator and the participants that my purpose in observing the class was to better learn about how people learn to give birth. The childbirth educator interacted with me throughout the course. She asked me clarifying questions, at times, about statistics and other data relating to maternal health. The hospital and the educator remain anonymous. Details concerning the course and the educator have been removed from this chapter in order to guarantee their privacy. I was not given permission to record audio of the class and relied on short-hand notetaking.

The childbirth education class my participant attended was at a local hospital in the Inland Empire; she later chose to give birth at the same hospital. In the labour and delivery ward at this particular hospital, 30 percent of patients have Caesarean sections. This rate, in comparison to the WHO's set standards for optimal healthcare is quite high. According to a medical professional from this hospital who was interviewed anonymously, the Caesarean sections actually hover at about 50 percent. "The labour and delivery board usually has at least half of the women prepping for a Caesarean section, regardless of what the actual data says," she told me in one interview. I asked how the data couldn't add up and she said that at times transfers from another hospital are not counted or emergency Caesarean sections will be relegated to a different statistic. Although this is anecdotal, I found that in interviewing other medical professionals at this hospital that many believed that half of the women who entered the doors of the labour and delivery ward left with a Caesarean section. With Caesarean sections hovering between 30 and 50 percent, I argue that this hospital must have set-up a standardized chare that polices the bodies—both mother and baby—into Caesarean sections. With that hypothesis made, I attended their free, open to the community, childbirth education course with my participant. I intended to see if my hypothesis could gather traction depending on how the childbirth education class created an environment of enabling physicality in labour or restricting movement. What kind of "conditioning," to use social scientist's Carrie Noland's term, do pregnant bodies undergo in this hospital-sponsored class? How does this class "police," to use performance studies scholar's Andre Lepecki's term the pregnant body? And lastly, how do pregnant people navigate the conditioning and policing and what kind of attempts of gaining agency over their birth experience erupt form their bodies in labour?

Case Study

I sat down in the back of the hospital's multipurpose room, watching couples—all heteronormative pairs—nervously chat with one another as they awaited the two-day hours-long lesson to begin. My participant showed up and decided to sit next to me as her partner was unable to make it to the first session. This was Susanna's second childbirth education course she had taken. She fervently pursed childbirth education so that she could make the most informed decision about where to and how to birth. At the time of the course, she was twenty-four weeks pregnant with her first child and humming with excitement over the idea of becoming a mother. Susanna grew up surrounded by a loving family in Mexico. She pursued higher education with the rest of her siblings in the United States. Her mother has seven children. Susanna happily recounted the story of her birth to me during our prenatal interview. She was a surprise twin! Her mother recounted that her birth was very painful and that she found out she was having twins when the doctor said, "Here comes another one!" Having a natural birth was important to Susanna, but not as important as having a healthy baby. She had attended one of her sister's births and witnessed her sister receive an episiotomy that later resulted in a laceration that ripped her sister's anal sphincter, which required surgeries in her first weeks as a mother. These social experiences arguably conditioned Susanna's body to first expect pain (from mother and sisters' birth stories) to expect that medical intervention can cause sever bodily trauma, and to see the body as a trickster. Her childbirth education class reinforced those concepts.

The childbirth educator began the course by standing at the podium in front of a PowerPoint screen. She introduced herself and her role at the hospital as both a nurse and educator, introduced me as a scholar in the room, and then began the class with exclaiming: "We're going to talk about pain. Pain that goes away ... but it will be the most painful experience of your life. Let's understand how we feel that pain and the effects of your stress, in feeling that pain, on your baby." If first-time mothers in that pale pink multipurpose room did not know much about birth, they certainly now knew that it was painful and that their own feeling of pain could potentially cause bodily harm to their baby. Although the opening words to this class did not have the pregnant participants participating in physical training, I argue that the impact of these words under the umbrella of education trains and conditions the body to expect a negative experience for both mother and baby. The prenatal interview I had with my participant, Susanna, after the class took place confirms my theory that the speech acts uttered in this childbirth education class help form a base of technique for childbearing women. In our interview, Susanna said the following to me: "I think that there's no way out of pain. I will be in pain. It's just a matter of how I will deal with the pain. It was helpful to have what I think was a contraction because it reminded me to start breathing. I needed to lie down. I hope that I'll be able to do that for twenty-four hours. No longer than that, though." Where did she learn to lie down during labour? Where did she learn that there was no way out of pain? Notice how Susanna is already saying that lying down through labour will help her through the pain. This conditioning, as I will continue to argue throughout this chapter, aids this particular hospital by ensuring compliancy and conformity from the patient. The couples in the room noticeably sank back into their chairs and all side conversation ceased. Compliancy begins.

The educator started an icebreaker by asking each couple to tell the room what their names are, their due date, the sex—conflated with gender—of their baby, whether they wanted to have an epidural, if they were going to breastfeed, and who their doctor was. This question to the participants sketches a score of normalcy—an epidural is the most common form of pain relief, breastfeeding is an option, and a doctor is probably going to attend your birth. The first attendant joyfully shared that she was having a girl. Smiles broke out all around the room, momentarily relieving the tension. She then shared that she was choosing to not have an epidural; her mother had her the natural way, so of course she could, too. The educator paused, put a hand on her hip and smiled. "You're saying no right now, right?" The attendant did not say anything in response. The childbirth educator continued to smile and said that is she wanted a natural birth, she should take Bradley childbirth education course or hire a doula, effectively reinforcing that nonmedicated vaginal birth is an alternative choice at this hospital and would need outside support. "You're saying no right now, right?" also conditions the mother to expect that medical interventions for pain relief will be necessary, regardless of the mother's birth plan or wishes. This is choreopolicing—the act of forming and "ensuring conformity" (Lepecki 9). The pregnant person, in this childbirth education class, is learning that her bodily autonomy can only function within the set structure of the medicalized industrial complex, yet she's also learning where she choreographs herself amidst this structure.

During the course a pregnant mother raised her hand and asked if she would be able to refuse any procedures, such as an episiotomy, during her birth experience at this hospital. The educator leaned on the podium and told her participants "you can refuse anything, but it may interfere with our time frame." In this hospital, there is a set choreographic score, a medical choreography, for how a birth experience should develop. This medical choreography imposes a reshaping of pregnant bodies from their autonomous state to a compliant and hopefully—in the eyes of the medical choreographer—docile labouring body.

The childbirth educator halfway through the course, quite out of the blue and without prompting from a question, shared a story that she found would be helpful to these first-time mothers and fathers. "Okay guys," she began, "I'm going to scare you." The participants shifted in their seats, and I noticed one mother turn her head into her partner's shoulder, as if not seeing the educator share this story would in some ways shield her pregnant body. "There is a serious risk when it comes to vaginal birth. If baby is at station -2 and ..." she said and looked over at me in the back of the room, and with a heavy sigh, she continued "Katie, we're talking about prolapsed cord." I nodded, unsure of my role but beginning to understand the role of this performance: to teach pregnant mothers and fathers about the wayward, tricky, and even deadly pregnant body. "One time," she continued, "I was doing a cervical check and yelled, 'I have a cord! Someone come in here!'" She smacked the podium and recounted her story, now yelling, "Dad! Hit the button!" The room became eerily quiet as the pregnant couples watched their educator. "Now, for prolapsed cord, you can bet that I don't move at all from here on out. I'm holding the baby's head as we're wheeled to OR for an emergency Caesarean section and during that entire operation." One brave participant raised her hand and asked how common a prolapsed cord occurrence was. "I'm not sure about the statistics, but I can tell you that I've seen that happen twice. Can a prolapse cord happen when you're walking around Target? Yes, yes it can." There was no nefarious purpose to these shared stories—the educator was obviously a caring, loving nurse. She was sharing what she had been taught and what she had witnessed as a labour and delivery nurse in a busy city hospital: women's bodies are othered form the self, and, at times, are uncontrollable and dangerous. These constructs do great harm to first-time pregnant mothers. Although the body can be a trickster and can be deadly, women have been having babies since time immemorial, and teaching them that the body can be deadly only promotes fear to ensure medical compliancy—the ultimate form of control in the hospital. And although a birthing body will do what it wants to and although any birth experience does not follow the proposed birth plan because of the body's unruliness, the effective choreopolicing set in place by the hospital in this example ensures conformity and compliancy and that itself is effective bodily training.

On the second day of the childbirth education course, I noticed that a few of the couples did not return. Was it due to the scare tactics? Or perhaps work or familial obligations? My participant, Susanna, returned with her partner and was looking forward to learning more about birth. The educator began the course and away we went learning about different ways to birth, what's allowed and not allowed, and what kind of births this particular nurse had experienced. When we got to the diagrams of the cervix dilated to 10cm in preparation for baby's birth, the educator said that there could be an issue, even if fully dilated. "If baby's head is bigger than the pelvis, then that's a major, major emergency" she exclaimed. "We'll try to deliver one shoulder first, but if we go to surgery, I honestly don't know what they'll do" she said quietly and shrugged her shoulders. She bit her lip and seemed to struggle with the decision to say the next part of her story. Clearing her throat, she continued, "One time, I heard that the head ... well ... that a baby got decapitated." Silence descended in the hospital's multipurpose room. I looked over at my participant and she seemed unfazed. I looked over to the doula across the way—who was taking this class as part of keeping her training up to date—witnessed her comforting a pregnant person next to her who started to cry. The educator attempted to comfort her audience by saying, "And there's no way of knowing that that will happen unless you even try to push. But, I don't want to scare you." Some participants were like the participant seated next to me: unfazed, prepared to learn more. Others were horrified to learn a body could do this, but can it? Was this just a tale she had heard among nurses? What was the purpose of telling this tale to pregnant couples? In essence, its purpose was to teach the pregnant body that it has no control or autonomy and that although the doctors are the medical choreographers of birth, sometimes they cannot save a baby from a murderous, pregnant body. And although this can all be prevented by having a planned Caesarean section—and here we start to comprehend why this particular hospital's Caesarean section rate is abnormally high—pregnant people are taught that their bodies during a normal vaginal birth can kill their babies. Trust should be placed in the hands of the medical professional and the pregnant body, according to the educator.

Performatively, the educator's talk lingers with me, as if her lesson held some key to why women in the U.S. are policed into unnecessary Caesarean sections. Although Lepecki would argue that "it is the dancer who, in the most policed, controlled spaces (say even in the tightest of choreographic scores), who has the potential to activate the appearing not necessarily of a subject" and "demonstrates that someone always finds a way to move politically" (20). How do women in these "tight" medical scores find a way to move politically?

It is too convenient to argue that women are simply policed into Caesarean sections at this hospital through the vehicle of childbirth education. Rather, I argue that the purpose of medical choreography is to implement certain kinds of movements from the pregnant person and to veto others to meet the needs of a for-profit industry. The pregnant person, though navigating these tightly policed spaces, always has the potential to find a way to move their body, and access the choreopolitical—the ability to know how to and to move freely. Even though the discourse in childbirth scholarship focuses on how the medical industrial complex shapes pregnant and childbearing women, in these childbirth education classes, pregnant women can gain knowledge as to how they will be policed; thus, they can prepare themselves for the medical choreography that awaits them should they choose this hospital. Susanna was happy to hear the stories of trauma and loss the educator shared. She told me that she wants to know as much as possible about everything that can go wrong so that she may prepare herself. Susanna is aware that things go wrong and wished to gain as much intellectual knowledge about birth before she had her baby. Robbie Davis-Floyd has written that pregnant women "equate knowledge with information" and "place their trust in intellectual knowledge, and not in intuitive, emotional, or bodily knowledge" (Davis-Floyd 31). To know is to control, and what better way to activate control over a wayward pregnant body than to attend multiple childbirth education classes as Susanna did?

Yet Susanna did much more than attend childbirth education classes; she also practised moving on a birthing ball from watching a video on YouTube, hired a doula, and when the time came for her daughter's birth, she practised breathing techniques she learned as an advanced dancer. She found the fissures and cracks in medical choreographies and pressed hard—training her body and gathering support through a doula. In her prenatal interview she shared the following:

> I want to be able to breathe through the pain without getting to the hospital and getting hooked up to an epidural. I also have food anxiety. I don't want to go to the hospital and eat ice chips.

> And, I read a paragraph in *What to Expect When You're Expecting* about doulas, something about your labour being shorter if you hire one.

Does Susanna prefer intellectual knowledge over other forms of knowledge, as Davis-Floyd would argue? No, she does not. As with many other women under U.S. maternal healthcare, she understands medical choreography and responds to it agentively, drawing on her own physical, intellectual, and emotional repertoires.

In our postpartum interview, I asked what helped the most in labour before she received an epidural for medical pain relief, and Susanna said that her breathing from her previous dance training. Although she might have sought intellectual knowledge from many different sources prior to the birth, she drew upon her experience as a dancer, and her body drew upon that experience in labour. Thus, what is happening here is more complicated than more policing resulting in higher Caesarean section rates. Susanna said that though she thought lying down in labour would help, she never did lie down:

> I was doing exercises, breathing. I would bounce and rock on the ball, left, right, and forward. The nurse would come in and fix the external fetal monitor if I dislodged it while I was on the ball. It was never a problem for me to be on the ball. Whenever I had a contraction the doula would tell me to relax my face, if I scrunched my face the rest of my body would contract. I did what I wanted to do, but I didn't limit myself. I didn't take any birthing classes besides the childbirth education class I took. A week before my due date, I went online and looked at different ways I could use a birthing ball. Everything I was doing in the hospital I had already practiced at home every day the week before. I watched YouTube videos about the birthing ball to accelerate labour. Rocking, bouncing, hugging it knees down. At some point I was squatting and trying to relax by the counter.

Susanna moved and activated the political by choreographing her own labour. Instead of lying down as instructed through childbirth education, she bounced and rocked and found her own way to dance on the boundaries of standardized care. Although she was not sure what to expect, she did not limit herself; she mobilized her body and her baby's body to create her own path for their childbirth experience. She had a plan, although the plan did not go as she wished it. Her unruly childbearing body and medical choreographies wrote a new score:

> The plan was for me to be able to withstand all that without pain medication. Also, I forgot to tell you that the nurse told me that those kicks I was feeling were contractions during my ultrasound. This is my first baby, so I didn't know that what I had been having were contractions—I just thought they were stronger kicks than usual. I went to the hospital to get checked out, but not thinking I'd have to stay.
>
> At 6PM, the on-call doctor came in, she checked my dilation at 6cm, she broke my waters. It was like a big needle that she broke my waters with. It was sad, because my amniotic fluid was already running super low so it was like peeing on myself. It was only like a quarter of a cup. It was nothing. I felt it on my butt and it was nothing. After that, they put the catheter in. Why did they put it in?

I asked Susanna if they asked her if it was okay to break her waters. She did not remember at the time of the interview. In the childbirth education course we attended, breaking waters was mentioned as a way to speed up labour. Susanna understood the medical choreographies at play and she saw nothing out of the ordinary with the doctor breaking her waters. Here, the medical choreographies of this hospital begin to close in on her own birthing choreographic endeavours. The nurse put a catheter in without asking for her permission. A catheter is normally inserted into the urethra when a patient is about to undergo an epidural or surgery. Susanna did not plan on having either. The catheter is essentially a tether to a pole for a childbearing body; it is one of the most restrictive techniques medical professionals can use to manipulate how the childbearing person can move in labour when there is no necessary reason for placing it. Why did she accept the catheter and the breaking of waters when both were unnecessary? Birthing classes can effectively train a pregnant body to be prepared for medical policing and to not have full control over their own bodily autonomy, which is what happened during Susanna's birth. She knew not to question what the doctor and nurses wanted to do with her body.

Susanna felt a loss of control. Her body started acting differently after her waters were broken:

> Oh, after the doctor broke my waters I started having the "non-baby," real contractions and it was bad. I felt heat, it was like fire. I felt heat on my hips, my pelvis, my vagina, my uterus, my everything—like fire, very hot. It was a pain I had never felt before. I was sobbing and yelling. Within minutes I started having the real contractions and it was unbearable. I stopped breathing. I couldn't breathe. It was bad. Everything the doula was asking me to do—I couldn't do it. She tried anything but nothing worked. She tried to put me in different positions and I didn't want to move. I was kneeling on the bed and hugging the back part of the bed. The nurses left me alone, they let the doula do the work. They even offered us a yoga ball because my doula's ball was deflated. The nurses would come in every five minutes and would never tell me to not move. When I had the catheter in, I was stuck on the bed but I could still move on it. She'd tell me to take a deep breath when I felt a contraction but I was like—HUH UH HUH UH HUH. It was so unbearable. I couldn't stop clenching my fist. It was a little bit past six when I asked for the epidural. Maybe I felt like it was a long time but I think it was only thirty minutes. That time I was yelling. You know you hear women yelling like crazy in the movies? That was me. I was like "HAAAA! HAAAA! HAAAA! I need pain relief!!!" I told the anesthesiologist to "go low-key on the epidural" because I didn't want to tear like my sister. It was not good because I felt a lot of vaginal pressure. It was not pain, it was pressure. It felt like I had to poop.
>
> At a little past seven, the doctor came in and said, "You are 9cm." Within the hour of my waters breaking, I dilated to 9cm. The doctor said, "I'm a little bit worried because your baby's heartrate is decelerating every time you're having a contraction." She's seeing that on the monitors. My baby's heart rate was going down to eighty, but never went where it was supposed to be at 110. She said, "Okay, we're going to try to push because you are not fully effaced and your baby's at station -1. We're going to do some practice pushes before we think about a C-section." So I

> pushed in sections. I would push for ten seconds and then rest, then push again for ten seconds. She checked the monitor to see how my baby's heart was doing and it wasn't working out. So she thought about it, and discussed it with me, so it wasn't working out for the baby, so that's when she decided ... or she recommended, that I should have a C-section. "I don't think your baby's going to be able to take the stress of natural labour." I said okay. But I cried so much because I had been in labour for more than forty-eight hours, and I felt a little devastated. I was very afraid that something was going to happen to my baby that I did what the doctor said. I was okay with the decision but it could have been better. I think that there's nothing that I can control concerning my daughter's stress level during labour. If she wouldn't have had a heart deceleration then I could have had a natural birth. I am very happy that the doula kept my stress level down and in that manner, my daughter's stress level. I feel like I survived because I paid attention to my body. I am a survivor. I am a survivor of labour.

Several troubling statements come out of Susanna's birth story. I opened this chapter with the educator telling her participants that the childbirth education class would focus on how a mother's pain can affect her baby. Susanna said there was nothing she could have done to controll her daughter's stress and compromised heart rate, yet a moment later, she said, "I am happy that the doula kept my stress level down and in that manner, my daughter's stress level." No matter how many times she told herself that she was not in control of her daughter's compromised heart rate, she still believed that she had some aspect of control, which connects this feeling to the childbirth educator's framing of the course as managing mother's body so it does not hurt baby. Although Susanna knew she was not responsible, she still wondered, and that seed of doubt in her body was placed by the childbirth education class. Susanna also shared that she was "very afraid that something was going to happen to my baby that I did what the doctor said." Where did she learn to fear? I contend that this particular fear had everything to do with learning that a woman's body is capable of murdering her baby, as she was taught in childbirth education class. How can a woman birth without that worry when she has the image of a decapitated baby in her head and inscribed into her body? Lastly,

Susanna's pain noticeably went up after the interventions of the breaking of the waters and the placement of the catheter. Although she tried to keep moving, with the encouragement of her doula, the pain eclipsed all attempts. Arguably, these interventions set the cascade toward a Cesarean section for Susanna. Not asking for her consent or explaining the risks to said interventions "de-mobilized political action by means of implementing a certain kind of movement that prevents any formation and expression of the political" (Lepecki 20). The hook to the waters and the needle to the urethra demobilized Susanna, and although she scored her own birth, she could not fully perform her plan due to the sweepingly powerful medical choreographies enacted on her body and her baby's body.

At the onset of this chapter, I asked how does a childbearing woman learn the technique of submission to medical authority prior to childbirth. In other words, how do pregnant women learn to have their childbearing bodies policed, ensuring conformity to the medical industrial complex? How do they then navigate these tight spaces of control—medical choreographies—to create their own choreographies of birth? I argue that childbirth education, especially hospital-sponsored community classes can demobilize a childbearing woman's bodily autonomy and teach a pregnant body to be prepared to be policed by medical authority and to expect to not have full control over their own bodily autonomy, which was evident Susanna's recounting of her birth. Hospital-sponsored childbirth education classes play a large role in training the pregnant body to expect pain and to expect their body to be dangerous to the baby. These medical choreographies are difficult to learn and to navigate in labour. Although there is the potential for women to become birth choreographers themselves—mobilizing movement as political action and finding fissures and cracks within the seemingly ironclad medical choreographies—it as an uphill climb.

Endnote

1 The Inland Empire is a region covering more than 27,000 square miles of Southern California. The region is home to Riverside and San Bernardino counties which have a combined population of four million. The city of Riverside, where this specific case study takes place, is twelfth largest city in California. Riverside itself was

established in the late nineteenth century and is infamously known as the citrus capital of the world. Riverside's first hospital opened in 1893, ten years after the city's official incorporation. Hospitals in Riverside County all provide free or affordable prenatal education. Caesarean section rates at these currently hospitals vary between 29 and 32 percent. In Riverside County, preterm birth rates range between 8.5 and 9.5 percent, within average of the state's 8.8 percent preterm birth rate (Joynt 25). The total average cost of a vaginal birth in the Inland Empire is $11,292, with the patient paying around $1,324; for Caesarean births, the average cost is $16,270, with the patient paying around $1,806 (42).

Works Cited

Joynt, Jen. "California Health Care Almanac: Maternity Care in California, Delivering the Data." California Healthcare Association, 2016.

Carter S.K. "Beyond Control: Body and Self in Women's Childbearing Narratives." *Sociology of Health & Illness*, vol. 32, no. 7, 2010, pp. 993-1009.

"Childbirth Education Classes: Types and Benefits." *American Pregnancy Association*, 2012, americanpregnancy.org/labor-and-birth/childbirth-education-classes/. Accessed 24 July 2018.

Davis-Floyd, Robbie. *Birth as an American Rite of Passage*. University of California Press, 2003.

Kraut, Anthea. *Choreographing the Folk: The Dance Stagings of Zora Neale Hurston*. University of Minnesota Press, 2008.

Lepecki, Andre. "Choreopolice and Choreopolitics: Or, the Task of the Dancer." *TDR/The Drama Review TDR/The Drama Review*, vol. 57, no. 4, 2013, pp. 13-27.

Marin, Deanna, et al. "Childbirth Expectations and Sources of Information Among Low- and Moderate- Income Nulliparous Pregnant Women." *Journal of Perinatal Education*, vol. 22, no. 2, 2006, pp. 103-12.

Noland, Carrie. *Agency and Embodiment: Performing Gestures/producing Culture*. Harvard University Press, 2009.

Pollock, Della. *Telling Bodies Performing Birth: Everyday Narratives of Childbirth*. Columbia University Press, 1999.

Notes on Contributors

Megan Davidson, PhD, is a Brooklyn-based labour and postpartum doula who has attended about 550 births and assisted over 1200 families postpartum. Her research interests include sexed bodies and gender identities, reproduction and procreation, fatphobia and body positivity, the expertise of doulas, and activism and social change.

Jessica Elbert Decker is Associate Professor of philosophy at California State University, San Marcos, and teaches in the philosophy, women's studies, and environmental studies departments. Her work has been published in *philosophia: a feminist journal, Epoche: a journal for the history of philosophy*, and *The Journal of the History of Sexuality*. Decker's current research examines the portrayal of female figures in Ancient Greek philosophy and mythology in order to interrogate the symbolic structures of patriarchy as they appear in Ancient Greek thought and psychoanalysis.

Alys Einion is associate professor of midwifery and reproductive health at Swansea University, Wales, UK. She gained her PhD from Aberystwyth University, where she studied women's narratives, the boundaries between fiction and nonfiction, and writing about sexual violence. She is a prolific writer and an equality activist. She is currently working with narrative representations of pregnancy and childbirth, hypnobirthing, midwifery identity, and self-storying. She is also a novelist, and writes provocative and gripping fiction from women's perspectives.

Erynne M. Gilpin is a Michif (Saulteaux-Cree Métis) PhD candidate with of Indigenous Governance at the University of Victoria. Her research examines Indigenous womxn's leadership, embodied governance and Land/Water based wellness and well-being practices. She also works as an Indigenous birth-doula and supports families in the birthing of their Nations on their home territories within cultural context.

Claire Marguerite Leonard Horn is a PhD candidate in law and graduate teaching assistant at Birkbeck University, London. She completed her MA in gender and legal studies at New York University, and her BA in English literature at McGill University. Her research interests include reproductive technologies, bioethics, and feminist critical legal studies.

Rebecca Howes-Mischel is an associate professor of anthropology at James Madison University; she received her PhD in cultural anthropology from New York University. She has conducted ethnographic research about gender, embodiment, and reproductive politics in Oaxaca, Mexico, and the United States.

Carla Ionescu researches the influential nature of Artemis both in the Greek world and in Ephesus. Her work provides evidence suggesting Artemis is the most prevalent and influential goddess of the Mediterranean, with roots embedded in the community and culture of this area, which can be traced further back in time than even the arrival of the Greeks.

Sarah Lewin, LMSW, is a New York based labour doula and Anthropology graduate student at The New School for Social Research. Sarah is interested in the intersection of personal and public dialogues around health, weight, and identity.

Catherine Ma is an associate professor of psychology at Kingsborough Community College. She received her Ph.D. from The Graduate Center of the City University of New York in social-personality psychology. Having experienced every single problem related to nursing her three children, she was inspired to use her research expertise to help women nurse their babies in an empowering manner and make informed decisions regarding infant feeding. Her research expertise focuses on breastfeeding ideology, the lived experiences of women, race and class in travel basketball, and the psychology of immigration.

Laura Major, PhD, is head of the English Department at Achva College in Israel. Besides her interest in English-language education, she is also fascinated by women's poetry, especially as it concerns the body. Other research interests include Holocaust literature, African women's literature, and pedagogical literature.

Maxime Polleri is a doctoral candidate in anthropology at York University and a MacArthur Nuclear Security pre-doctoral fellow in the Center for International Security and Cooperation at Stanford University. His former area of interest explored the aesthetics of kawaii, an ideal that advocates cuteness and childish behavior among Japanese women. As a 2015-2016 fellow of the Japan Foundation and doctoral fellow of the Canadian Social Sciences and Humanities Research Council, he researched the Fukushima Daiichi nuclear disaster, with a particular emphasis on the problem of radioactive contamination.

Jen Rinaldi is an assistant professor in the legal studies program at the University of Ontario Institute of Technology. She earned a doctoral degree in critical disability studies at York University, where she researched how disability diagnostic technologies affect reproductive decision making. Currently, she engages with narrative and arts-based methodologies to deconstruct eating disorder recovery and to story traumatic histories of institutionalization.

Katie Nicole Stahl-Kovell is a feminist ethnographer and dance scholar of childbirth and maternal embodiments. She employs both critical feminist ethnography and dance studies as social theory in her work as scholar and activist to explore the intersections between embodied knowledges and systems of power. Stahl-Kovell is currently working on her dissertation, *Choreographing Childbirth*, as a PhD candidate of critical dance studies at the University of California, Riverside. Through ethnography of pregnancy, childbirth education, and live labours, she untangles epistemologies and performances of childbirth. Katie is a Dean's Distinguished Fellow, Gluck Fellow of the Arts, and holds a MA in Southeast Asian studies from UC Riverside; she is also McNair Scholar in anthropology from CSU Dominguez Hills.

Karen Walasek, MFA, MEd, is a mother, grandmother, artist, and former midwife. She is currently a doctoral candidate in sustainability education at Prescott College where she focuses on the intersection between motherhood studies, decolonization practices and narrative inquiry.

Ruchika Wason Singh has pursued her creative interests she completed a BFA in 1997 and a MFA in 1999 from College of Art, New Delhi. In 2001, she undertook a research project on the sociological frameworks within Indian colonial and postcolonial art at University of Delhi. She received her PhD in 2008.

Sarah Marie Wiebe grew up on Coast Salish territory in British Columbia, BC, and now lives in Honolulu, HI. She is an assistant professor in the Department of Political Science at the University of Hawai'i, Mānoa, where she focuses on environmental sustainability. Her book *Everyday Exposure: Indigenous Mobilization and Environmental Justice in Canada's Chemical Valley* (2016) with UBC Press won the Charles Taylor Book Award (2017); it examines policy responses to the impact of pollution on the Aamjiwnaang First Nation's environmental health. At the intersections of environmental justice and citizen engagement, her teaching and research interests emphasize political ecology, participatory policymaking, and deliberative dialogue.